THE TROUBLED DEEP

THE TROUBLED DEEP

by Rob Parker

To Tim,

All my very best,

R A V E N 🐦 B O O K S

LONDON · OXFORD · NEW YORK · NEW DELHI · SYDNEY

RAVEN BOOKS
Bloomsbury Publishing Plc
50 Bedford Square, London, WC1B 3DP, UK
29 Earlsfort Terrace, Dublin 2, Ireland

BLOOMSBURY, RAVEN BOOKS and the Raven Books logo
are trademarks of Bloomsbury Publishing Plc

First published in Great Britain 2025

A catalogue record for this book is available from the British Library.

ISBN: HB: 978-1-5266-8190-4; TPB: 978-1-5266-8191-1;
EBOOK: 978-1-5266-8186-7; EPDF: 978-1-5266-8187-4

2 4 6 8 10 9 7 5 3 1

Typeset by Integra Software Services Pvt. Ltd.
Printed and bound in Great Britain by CPI Group (UK) Ltd, Croydon CR0 4YY

MIX
Paper | Supporting
responsible forestry
FSC
www.fsc.org
FSC® C171272

To find out more about our authors and books visit www.bloomsbury.com
and sign up for our newsletters

For Becky, always.

And for my family, without whom I'd be nowhere.

November 1987

Mum and Dad really like parties. They go to three or four a week sometimes, but we are never allowed to go with them. Me and my big brother, that is. They say it's because the parties always finish too late. That there are no party games, no ice cream, no musical statues. That we'd be home too late for school the next day.

They are probably right about this, but that doesn't mean I don't want to go. Getting all dressed up the way Mum does in her sparkly frocks and jangling earrings. My brother could get cleaned up like Dad does too, handsome in a suit or a leather jacket. Mum and Dad always look so special as we wave from the window, watching them leave Brindley Hall in their super cool Jaguar car.

Dad taught me an old-timey rhyme about it and I like the way it rolls off the tongue. *Father's car is a jaguar, and pa drives rather fast.* I am going to tell the other children at school on Monday.

If I get to school on Monday.

Because tonight, it has all been different. This time, when it went dark, the babysitter didn't come, and Mum told us both to get dressed smartly instead. This time, we got to go with them in the Jaguar car, named after a big cat, because it goes so fast.

I wish it had been faster. I wish we'd gone far away from here.

I wish it hadn't gone into the water.

I wish I wasn't stuck in it, me and my brother looking at each other in the back as freezing water comes up through gaps in the floor.

I wish we were at home.

I wish we'd never gone to that party.

I

The silence woke him.

Just as it did every night.

It somehow seemed cacophonous, with a mind and drive all its own. It gripped him with noiseless compression so that it felt as if the bones of his head wanted to meet in the middle, his brain in between be damned.

It wanted Cameron Killick to suffer.

He grasped at his hair to try to stop it, but as the crush became almost too great, there was a whining sound, like a split valve. The pressure released, just a fraction. He cracked open his eyes as the lifting pain allowed his lids movement.

Nala, his dog, was right there above him. Licking his cheek. That whine was hers. Seeing her eyes, earnest marbles of dark chocolate, pulled him out of the vice.

He reached up to stroke her behind the ears.

'Thank you,' he whispered.

Another night, another attack. Assaulted by silence, which released the dogs of old horrors into his subconscious. They tore through him, untethered, until they caused a full-scale siege of panic.

He got out of bed, the sweat rolling off him and landing with dotting spatters on the hardwood floor of his bedroom. Entering the bathroom, he turned on the taps and waited in the dark as the bath filled with tepid water.

Was it getting worse? Or was this better? He had no idea anymore. All he could do was keep ticking onward, day by day.

Nala jumped up onto the tiled countertop next to the bath and got comfortable while he lowered himself in. The snorkel was already there, and he put it into his mouth, blew it clear, then shut his eyes and lay back. Submerging himself fully, Cam breathed deeply.

In for a count of three.

Hold for five.

Out for eight.

And slowly, with the myriad minutiae of life above the surface muffled by the water, he could have thoughts that were his own again. His muscles began to uncoil, his shoulders soon flat against the bottom of the tub.

PTSD. Acute.

He could hear the bullets, even when they weren't actually flying.

But underwater, he never heard a thing.

So Cam Killick lay there, with Nala on watch, neither of them asleep nor awake, until daybreak.

2

Cam watched the dawn mist lift off the wheat field, a sea of frozen stalks in front of him – except for a few that waved as Nala brushed past. She raced through the crop as he walked around its perimeter on the old farm track that led back up to his home. He felt the drugs course through his system – the daily cocktail he had to take to keep from tumbling further into himself – and the gnarled edges of his nerves seemed to smooth further with every passing second.

He had only just turned forty, and the constant lack of good sleep was gradually getting to him, leaving a permanent mental fog. He lived on what felt like half-speed, guided by a jaded autopilot with tar-like instincts.

Nala appeared at his side. She looked up at him for approval, appreciation, agreement, any and all of the above. He nodded at her, and she darted off again, the wobbling wheat kernels the only indication of her route. She had been jet black when he'd got her as a pup a couple of years ago. Now, aged almost three, she was the colour of gun smoke. A Shih Tzu-Yorkshire terrier cross, she needed these early explosions of activity – they calmed her for the rest of the day. She was the only sentient creature Cam had let close to him in years.

As he wound to the end of the farm track, scuffing the loose stones of a roadway long since eroded, he pulled out his phone and checked the weather app. Not the commercial ones like the BBC or Sky – he got his data direct from the Meteorological Office. The same way the military did. They rarely got things wrong, and if it wasn't broke, he wasn't going to attempt to fix it.

Little sunshine symbols, fringed by white cloud. The conditions were going to be perfect. The air felt good, too. It was crisp, but not cold.

He wanted to get going. He felt the pull of the water, out there somewhere. And of what he might find in its depths. The heft and draw of the Brindley mystery sat heavy around his shoulders. His head and heart both pulsed with it, and he ran through the bullet points of his plan as he walked.

Go to the site he'd earmarked for today.

Check with sonar.

If something appeared, get down there. Confirm it.

If it's a jackpot, call the police.

The track they took for their usual walk had only a couple of buildings along its stretch, ending in a secluded farm. It was a public right of way up to the farm gate, while the fields either side were also the farm's. The owner paid no attention to the quiet loner who walked up and down it twice a day, at dawn and dusk. Now he was on his way back home, to get started on the day.

Cam's home, Haven Cottage, a small barn conversion near the village of Neatishead, rose above the hedgerows and haze ahead of them. The original stone mass had been put there some century and a half ago, and the renovation into a dwelling happened only three decades back. It was nicely appointed, but no good for families, and he had heard it used to be a long-term conundrum for local rental companies. For him, however, it was perfect, so he bought it outright – the ideal thing to spend his military pension on.

Having a pension before you hit forty. Now that was a thing.

Pension suggested retirement. The sedentary. A winding down. He wanted none of those things, only the quiet so often associated with them.

Haven Cottage was tight to the farm track, thrust up close to the hedge, rendering the downstairs windows with a close view of English holly and very little else – even daylight. It also meant that any parking was round the side, in a stone yard that used to be for the ploughs to turn around in. His van was there, nose pointed out, ready to go. A navy Volkswagen T5 Transporter with everything stripped out save for the front two captain seats. One for him, one for his canine co-pilot. Another gift from his military pension, although he had used the PTSD compensation payout for that one.

'Go on,' he said to Nala, unclipping her lead as they entered the yard. She trotted to the passenger door of the van. She didn't even need to duck as he opened it, and she hopped up the step and into the footwell, where food and a water bowl were waiting. She turned and looked at him with a forlorn expression.

'We're getting something on the way, don't worry,' he told her, and shut the door. He rounded the van, taking one last look at the sky, then climbed in behind the steering wheel.

The van was very full. The walls on both sides, save for the sliding door behind the passenger, had been stripped back, replaced by wooden boards against which shelving was fixed either side of a clear space to change in, full of neatly organised equipment. Diving masks, wetsuits, dry suits, gauges, regulators, rash vests, fins, hoods, sonar equipment, audio-visual gear, ropes and buoys. Along with his four air tanks, some full, some not. He left empty and almost-empty ones in his van, strapped to the racks, for his regular trips to the scuba store in Cromer to get his tanks refilled. Always good to get them refilled when passing.

It was a scuba store on wheels. All handpicked. Some of the gear was new and shining, while other pieces were battered and the more trusted for it. Experience had taught him that you never knew what you might need, so it was best to have it all just in case.

Twenty years' worth of remnants and teachings from an elite military diving career spent fighting water-bound adversaries and pulling all sorts up from the deep with the Special Boat Service. Everyone knew the Special Air Service, or the more pop-culture friendly SAS. But the SBS were every bit as daring. Every bit as elite. Only their battleground was water.

Everything was prepared. He turned back, satisfied, and left with a dieseled grumble, breaking the stillness of an erstwhile typical countryside morning. He was off – en route to the potential resting place of a decades-old mystery. And he couldn't get there quick enough.

3

Neatishead was arranged on the chicane of a country road, and Cam drove through its empty centre. A serene village, it had a couple of pubs, a shop and, on the outskirts, an astonishing decommissioned radar station. Its huge green mast stood tall over the surrounding tree tops an omnipresent reminder of the area's links to the Second World War. As Cam drove past it, he saw the chain-link fence was open, meaning it was one of those days in the year when tourists were welcome to visit. He looked through the gate – a view of a different era of service to his own – before pressing on deeper into the Norfolk Broads national park, heading for Potter Heigham.

There was a burger van there that did something called a 'bin lid barm' – a bread roll full of eggs, bacon, beans, cheese, black pudding, sausage and hash browns. Even forty-year-old cold cases could wait until after one of those had been factored in. He defied anyone to have a bad day after getting that down them. With the sun heading skywards, he pulled over to grab the breakfast, two coffees, a bottle of water and three extra loose sausages. Nala looked at the wrapped packages as he stashed them in the driver's door storage.

'No,' he said, stroking Nala's head, but she still looked up to lick his palm, desperate for any taste of whatever was hiding in those bags. Cam let her, and set off again, but not before popping two ibuprofen for the tension head-ache that had sat thumping in his head all morning like an obstinate toddler on the drums. His days almost always started this way, and on the rare occasions they didn't, he wondered why until he worried himself into another one.

The roads were getting busier, but only marginally. Life was more sedate in this part of the world, and that was why he loved it here. He had originally come to the region with work while his life was deteriorating and he was determined not to understand the root cause. A heli-copter had gone down in one of its many rivers, and he had been part of a salvage unit seconded to pull out the wreckage – and the dead.

He had got a taste for the area and the way the water felt when he was in it – dark, unpredictable, calming – and when he got out of the service, he came here on a more permanent basis. It allowed him to do the things he loved, in a place that inspired him, a world away from the blood-shed and danger he'd become so accustomed to.

He indicated left and took a turn between two thick hedgerows. The road wound tighter now, a single, narrow lane, and Cam took it slow and sensible, as usual. A lifetime spent ferrying around tanks of compressed air would do that to you. It wasn't the risk of the tanks breaking however; it was to prevent the valves from getting damaged. A valve that suddenly got loose would pinball around the inside of the van until it eventually ran out of air – or cannoned out through the windscreen.

The foliage got thicker on either side of the road. Cam began to see signs for Hickling Broad, which meant he was getting closer. It was round here somewhere, the turn-off. He knew it was.

Just as he wondered whether he had gone too far, he almost whizzed right by it, and had to brake hard to make the turn. He felt his teeth bare and heard a couple of soft metallic clunks behind him as the compressed air tanks in the back took the turn with him. He almost felt the tail wheels of the van begin to slip as they fought for purchase on the grass of the disused track, but the hardy vehicle fought well to keep straight.

And then he was there, between the trees in an overgrown tunnel of foliage, the branches and leaves reaching in on all sides. It was dark, a wormhole into the forest. Cam would have to be careful. He knew the water couldn't be far away. The maps of this part of the county were sketchy – literally, they had no more detail than a sketch. This 'road' was just that, a faded line on a decades-old map he'd got from the central library in Norwich some fifteen miles away.

'Hang on,' he said, as much to himself as to Nala. The branches raked at the flanks of the vehicle and Cam winced with every screech. It was tighter than he had anticipated, but its wildness gave him a good feeling about his objective. The more off-track, the better. He could feel it. The old buzz of excitement at getting close.

Every so often a stone column would appear, themselves near-swallowed by green on either side of the track. Cam smiled. Fence posts. The ground was getting softer, saturated with more water. But he couldn't see the actual body of Hickling Broad yet. He shouldn't be able to miss it: fifteen hundred acres of open water and marshland, the latter of which he had to concede he might already be in.

He slowed the van and got out, then got down on his haunches to press his hand to the earth. There was no water coming up between the blades of grass. It was still OK. He walked further down the track, trudging along in his three-quarter length dryrobe and wellies, assessing the feel with every step. He wouldn't want to race down here, but he could certainly inch the van along.

He went fifty metres, careful, eyes flitting from the spaces between trees down to the soaked earth, and back again. He could so easily make a wrong move and find himself sinking into a bog. The terrain was beautiful but fraught with potential peril, and with the residual head-ache still echoing through his head, it would be easy to make a dangerous error.

Up ahead, through a gap in the trees, he could see the ghostly shape of an abandoned wooden tower, with a small, broken turbine on its roof. He'd seen it on Google Earth. He was getting close.

At fifty metres in, the trees on the left parted, and the wild water yawned at him. He held his breath. New reed stalks littered the grass as it yielded to mud, then water. They had the haphazard distribution of nature in action. Those smaller saplings were natural reproduction, as opposed to something with a more human design. The woods were trying to reclaim the opening that had been thrust upon them, where the old boating track used to be.

This was the right place.

The water beckoned him over.

It looked untouched, perfect. The peat excavation that had been flooded to create the unique waterways of the Norfolk Broads dated right back to the twelfth century. By finding this spot, Cam felt he'd driven right into history.

He checked the ground one more time, made sure it would support the van. If anything, he felt it was somehow stronger further in. He ran back, his very synapses pulsing. Hopping in, Nala stared at him for an update. 'This is the spot, Nala. This is it.'

She span on the seat, a tight circle, as if sharing Cam's palpable excitement. He eased the vehicle along and pulled up at the gap, then checked the Met Office again for precipitation. The last thing he wanted was for a sudden torrential downpour, the kind that the British Isles was so adept at summoning on a whim, and for the track to become boggy. But the report read clear, and the sky, a firm grey-white like a heron's wing, looked set. He peered through the window at the water.

Hickling Broad carried an iconography in the pantheon of Norfolk myths and legends, with a unique, unforgiving character of its own. Only accessible via the river Thurne, through a sequence of cut-throughs and dykes, some of which were maintained and just about navigable, while some were not. It was remote, wild and self-perpetuating. The seasons rolled past in a zoetrope of colour change.

It appeared as good as any of the places he'd tried before.

No. It was *better*.

The perfect place for something to remain undiscovered for almost forty years.

4

He started the way he always did, with the small fold-out table, a water bowl and the bin lid barm. He let Nala out and told her to stay close. It was unnecessary, because when he put a sausage on a paper plate, he knew she'd be going nowhere else.

Between bites, Cam took out the bait caster fishing rod. With a three-pound test curve, it was capable of hauling in monsters. But Cam didn't keep such robust equipment for fishing. Instead of using the rod to pull things in, he used it to cast them out – namely a Bluetooth activated, Wi-Fi enabled sonar unit, weighing about half a pound. He took the orange bulb-shaped device and clipped it to the end of the line. Then came his phone and the sonar app. He connected the two devices, put the phone face up on the table, and cast as far as he could, out to the left-hand side of the visible water.

At the bottom of the screen appeared a wavy orange line, with a flat white line near the top. Linked up, with a strong reading.

Perfect.

He started to turn the reel, drawing the orange dot on the water gradually closer. While he did this, the image on the screen changed. Dots appeared in the middle, while the lower line went up and down. That was the bottom, and the numbers on the left detailed depth. Fifteen feet. Twelve feet. Sixteen feet.

Very changeable.

Soon, the numbers got smaller. Nine feet, seven feet, six feet. The sonar unit was closer to the bank now, and he continued pulling it in. Three feet. Two feet. One. With a rattle, the unit swung up out of the water and dangled below the tip of the rod.

He checked the screen and scrolled back along the entire reading, scouring the lower line.

He was looking for something different. Something strange, not made by the hands of nature. In this case, it would be a steep angle or a straight line. But there was nothing. Just the natural roll of silt and erosion that was commonplace in all the local waterways here.

He took a bite of his breakfast, and squeezed the knot between his shoulder blades, kneading it gradually looser. Steadying himself, he cast again, this time to a spot three feet to the right of his last cast. He repeated the process with the same attentiveness. Again, nothing. By doing this, he could cover the entirety of the water in front of him to a distance of about a hundred and fifty feet out.

On other jobs and other targets, he would ordinarily like to check the bottom further out than fifty metres, but he didn't think he needed to on this occasion.

When a car dropped into the water, it tended to stay put.

He repeated. And repeated. Calm, steady, methodical.

On the eighth cast, he saw something. A straight edge, three feet off the bottom, down to the bed at a shallow angle. He didn't jump to conclusions, but that size was a very good sign.

Could be a bonnet. Could be a boot. Could be an upended shopping trolley, too, but he decided to stay positive that answers, not just for himself but for the region at large, were coming.

He repeated the cast in the same place and reeled in slowly.

The line was there again, the drop off just as steep. But he could see slightly more this time. In his excitement, this second cast must have been off by a foot or so. Whatever it was, it was big.

His heart began to race, and with it came a sickly sweat. His breath came in sharp bursts as the excitement ramped up. When he looked at the sky, floaters danced in his vision.

He couldn't wait any more. He needed to get in the water.

'Nala, in or out?' he asked, walking back to the van. Nala looked at the water bowl, decided it wasn't as appealing as the food bowl Cam kept in the van at all times, and trotted to the passenger door. 'Good idea,' he said as she hopped in. He climbed in the back, suiting up in his five-millimetre wetsuit with hood and gloves. Fins and tank. Checked the regulators, checked the valves. All the while he was thinking about the story that brought him to this spot in the first place. The story that had somehow transfixed him.

The tale of the Brindley family.

How thirty-eight years ago, a family of four set off in their Jaguar XJ40 from a party in Norwich to drive back to their stately home deep in the Norfolk marshland, never to arrive. Like a mythical castle after its king's abdication, their estate tumbled to rack and ruin, and they were never seen again.

The parents of the quartet, Freddie and Maud, were big news. A glamorous couple, fuelled by the money made from his investment banking business. While he advised the country's high-and-mighty, she had brushed with the stars.

This particular night, they'd been at the party with their two children, Tommy and Hannah, who were eleven and seven at the time. The assembled press had waved them off with flashbulbs.

They weren't declared missing for a while. Everyone wasn't in everyone else's pockets back then, not like today with social media and phones beeping incessantly. After a fortnight, when Tommy and Hannah didn't reappear at school, the police started looking for them all, but their appeals amounted to nothing.

For a short time, the county went mad for the mystery. Norfolk had Brindley fever. But like any passing fad, interest waned. Many assumed after a while that the family had simply moved on; the theatricality of their sudden departure in keeping with the attention-seeking ways the parents were known for. As cold cases went, this one was Arctic.

Until Cam Killick heard about it three years ago on the *Norfolk Unexplained* podcast, which was a monthly digest of the county's most interesting unsolved mysteries. Then he had looked at a map of the area – and saw all that water.

Had anyone checked it at the time?

Cam became convinced that the Brindleys were under the surface of the Norfolk Broads somewhere – and was determined to find them.

The local police, for the most part, had thought he was mad. After a few cursory searches at the time, they simply didn't think there was any possible spot in the predominately shallow Norfolk Broads in which an entire saloon could stay hidden for forty years.

But they didn't know water. Not like Cam did. Cam had become devoted. He'd missed the drive and urgency of his previous life, and pouring himself into something as important as this took his attentions away from the fragilities and daily balancing acts of his mental state. It gave him a purpose. He'd become obsessed. The vacuum left by the end of his career, and the bitterness he'd felt about the manner of its ending, was filled by this self-imposed odyssey. He always felt, in those deep, subconscious pits of his, that if he found the Brindleys, he'd find himself again too.

And that was why, tugging his face mask on with a nod to Nala, he marched into the frigid waters of Hickling Broad – to the dark shape at the bottom, and all the grim secrets it could hold.

5

The water felt like jagged ice forced into his cells, but Cam knew he would soon acclimatise. As a point of personal habit, he always preferred dropping in as opposed to the gradual submersion of walking in step by step – it got the shock out of the way in a bone-jangling instant. But there was nowhere to do that here. Walking in like this, flippers in hand until he was out into open water, forced his body to experience the shock of the cold in increments. The toes, but that was over quickly. Then the knees, reminding him of every jumping jack and squat during those years of physical training. Then the family jewels, which let the entire body know just how unhappy they were with the drop in temperature.

Cam was used to all of this now, and his adrenaline and excitement acted as both a shield and personal heater. He was bursting to get beneath the surface.

Just before he did, he took stock of his position once more. Ahead, the water was vast, open to the elements and deathly quiet, ringed by swathes of bullrushes and reeds. It was an idyllic, picture-book example of the kind of vistas the Norfolk Broads were famous for. He turned back to where he'd come in from, and there, in the opening, was his van. Cam could just about make out the small dark shape of Nala's head in the passenger window, keeping eager watch.

Looking directly at the vehicle, he took a compass reading on his watch and made a mental note. It was more than just a compass or timepiece – it was a Suunto D6I dive computer that sat on his wrist and monitored his every trip. It fed him his dive time, his GPS position, the temperature – and most importantly – how much air was left in his tank. All this linked up to his computer in the van, to give him a full post-dive technical rundown of his time in the water.

Now, it told him the water temperature was eight degrees Celsius, or some forty-six degrees Fahrenheit.

Chilly.

As soon as the water was up to his chest, Cam reached down and tugged on his flippers, which multiplied his speed and manoeuvrability now that the water was deep enough. Suddenly free and moving, he lowered his head under the surface.

The quiet, underwater world calmed him within seconds. His headache lifted instantly, his heart pumping with a more dependable frequency and his brain cleared of all distraction. The silence was blissful.

Rejuvenated, emboldened and feeling almost electrically alive, he started swimming in the direction of the sonar shape.

Initially, he had to go off instinct and experience only because the visibility underwater was poor, swirling with sediment. He could see two or three feet in front of him at most. The water carried a brown tinge, with wide spokes of light pushing through in grey-white columns from the sky above.

Cam forged tentatively deeper, every kick laden with respect for the might of the water around him. And as he descended, the sediment was less disturbed by the wash created by the bank. The water was clearer, visibility now out to six feet. Below him, he could see the reaching tendrils of occasional weed clumps, and underneath, the earthen silt that caked the bottom of the broad, punctuated by the occasional stone.

Cam pressed deeper, keeping tight to the bottom, where it became dimmer by the second as less daylight could force its way down. With his stomach maybe a foot above the deck, he traced the decline into the murk.

It became darker still, and Cam was suddenly glad for the season. If he'd found this site in summer, he'd be hacking through thick knotweed. It may even have meant he couldn't dive at all and would have to sit on this tantalising knowledge for months. Thankfully, timings had aligned with mercy and favour.

All he needed now was to find it.

He reached for the torch on his belt, clicked it on, and a cone of light forged into the swirling murk.

Further. Deeper. Gradually, a foot at a time.

Until…

A spark up ahead. Some twelve feet away. No, not a spark – a glint. Cam passed his torch beam over the same spot. A bright dot bounced back, about three feet from the bottom. Taking it carefully, his heart clattering in his rib cage through excitement now rather than nerves, he edged closer. Almost savouring it. As a diver, spending so many hours in the mirthless, unforgiving subsurface world, these moments of discovery were what he lived for.

He held focus on that glint. A strip of something metallic. Then a dark shape around it. Larger, and dense. Cam held his breath. It took shape — a familiar one. Straight edges in a world that had none. A yellow square emerging in the low centre of it and black shapes on the square, becoming more legible by the second.

A number plate.

G472 RSM.

Cam felt a tremor around his knees as his torch scanned across the lettering.

This was it. Cam thought of all the years that had passed since this car had last been seen, and the weight of them made him almost dizzy.

This was it.

The thing they wrote books, made radio programmes about. What people speculated for decades over and swapped wild theories about.

Cam Killick had found it.

This, without doubt, was the Brindley car.

And the final resting place of the Brindley family.

September 1987

It feels like a hot summer day, even though I know winter is just around the corner. We are in the rowing boat on the lake next to Brindley Hall. Me, Dad and Tommy.

Mum is back in the house with some illness Dad's been calling a hangover. I don't know what it means. Mum just looks like she's got a headache and judging by the flushing of the toilet all morning, a tummy bug too.

Dad said it's the perfect day to go and see what's in the lake, and I know he means fish because he's brought a fishing rod along too, and a little pot that's got a lid on it.

The boat is dirty and came with the house. We've never been in it before and when it first hit the water, I was sure we were going to sink. We haven't got life jackets on, and I feel like Mum would want us to.

Dad is rowing us into the middle of the lake, one big pull after another, while me and Tommy sit on the bench at the back of the boat. I find it hard to sit still but I've got to keep my knees pressed together so they don't touch the cobwebs on the sides. I'm so excited, much more excited than Tommy I think, who looks like he'd rather still be inside. His blue eyes stare at the water like he's scared he might fall in.

'Here looks good,' Dad says, and pulls the oars back in the boat. They splash cold water on my legs. He drops a heavy weight on a rope over the side and ties it to the boat. 'There we are.'

It's strange and quiet being out on the water. Like nothing can get to us. The smell of the water is strange too, as if the colour green actually had a smell of its own. It's so quiet and it feels so weird that I can't help but blurt out a giggle.

Dad smiles. 'Now, now,' he says in a loud whisper. 'Don't make so much noise, or the fish will swim away.'

'Where are they Dad?' I ask, copying his hushed talking.

'Right underneath us, if we're lucky!'

I look down at the old wooden boards that make up the floor of the rowboat, in total wonder that they are the only thing separating us from where the fish are living right this second. I think of them darting about like silver arrows. The excitement surges up from my tummy.

'Are we going to catch them?' I ask.

'We are going to try,' Dad says, and he picks up the fishing rod. 'Tommy, could you get me a couple of maggots please?'

He hands Tommy the little pot. *What on earth are maggots?*

'Just open the lid carefully and take a couple out,' Dad says, still smiling.

Tommy gently peels open the tub and looks inside. 'Ugh!' he says, holding them back out to Dad.

'Maggots,' Dad says, taking them from Tommy and holding them out. 'They're the babies of flies.' He takes the lid off, and what is inside is so disgusting I can't stop looking at it. It's full of little pink bogeys that won't stop wriggling. 'You put them on the hook, and the fish come to eat them. That's how you catch them. Do you want to get two for me, Tommy?'

Tommy looks like he might be sick.

'I'll do it!' I say.

Dad smiles. 'OK, only if you want to. Gently now, with your fingers.'

'Sorry, Dad,' says Tommy.

Dad ruffles Tommy's hair. 'It's all right, son. You don't have to do anything you don't want to do.'

Carefully, I reach forward and dip my fingers into the pot. It's so much softer than I thought it was going to be and warm, somehow. It tickles too, and I can't help it, I giggle again. 'Got one!' I squeak.

'Perfect.' Dad takes it from me and pushes a hook through it. The maggot wriggles like crazy and suddenly I stop giggling. I don't know how I feel about it anymore.

'OK,' Dad says, before he tosses the maggot over the side and flicks the rod out into the water. A little red blob appears. 'That's the float,' he says. 'When it goes under, it means we've got a fish.'

I stare at the little red blob and listen to the birds and the breeze in the trees. The blob seems to go up and down with the little waves the wind makes on the water.

Nobody says anything – until suddenly, the float slides underwater and Dad springs into action, lifting his rod high. There's some splashing, then suddenly, lying on the surface next to the boat is a slab of silver with bright orange eyes.

'Wow,' Dad says. 'That's a good start!'

'What is it?' Tommy asks.

'A roach. Nice one too! I don't suppose they've ever been fished for before.'

A voice comes from the bank. 'Freddie? Freddie!'

All three of us turn to look at Mum, standing on the water's edge in her dressing gown.

'It's the phone,' she shouts. 'It's urgent.'

'OK, we're coming.'

Dad looks sad. I know I'm sad. I'm so fed up of the phone ringing. It's always work, work, work. When I'm grown up, I'm never going to have a job, so nobody can chase me with a phone all day. I'm just glad it's not attached to him, in his pocket or something. That would be *awful*.

'Thanks for taking us fishing, Dad,' I say.

He smiles at me, and I know he means it. 'You're welcome, darling.'

6

Breathe, Cam. *Breathe.*

He forced himself to swallow a lungful, right down to his stomach, then blew it out slowly – all the while staring at that number plate, thinking how he was the first to lay eyes on it in over three decades.

Another breath.

Get back to process.

First thing? Mark it. From his belt, he unclipped a length of thin rope with a hook on one end and what looked like an orange balloon on the other. With a pull of the toggle, it inflated to the size of a football. He planted his feet on the bottom and stepped forward, careful not to trip on his fins.

The car revealed more of itself with every step. Jesus. *Jesus.*

It was their car all right. A classic Jaguar XJ luxury saloon in countryside-green, hammered by the seasons and the continuous cyclic nature of inland aquatic ecology. The once-silver hubcaps were now a mucky brown, the tyres themselves half-swallowed by the eager silt. The windows were thick with accumulated sediment, the lustre of the chrome detailing pocked with rust chunks.

The body work however was OK, the soft green colour of it holding firm against the pressures of the environment. *The bonuses of a freshwater resting place*, Cam thought. Everything survived better when not submerged in the salt of the punishing sea.

Placing his hand on the back bumper, the car's place in history seemed to hit him all at once. Answers were coming at last.

He took the metal hook, reached under the bumper itself, and attached it under the vehicle. It would hold. He then released slack, glancing upwards at the surface, until the balloon broke through the rolling meniscus and into the morning air.

He looked through the water to the sky above and the world he'd come from moments earlier – a place where this car was still lost to history. Yet down here, in the muffled solitude and comforting pressure of the underwater, history had revealed itself to him. The thrill was thick and pulsing.

Bringing his wrist up, Cam checked the readings on his watch. He clicked a few buttons and set a GPS marker. He wasn't losing this place. Not now.

He took another two deep breaths. The water seemed to drop a couple of degrees, as the warmth of discovery gave way to a pure dread. Looking at the vehicle and those grimy windows, he knew he would have to face its contents.

The human side of this mystery had been the principal reason he'd carried on searching for so long. Because of the puzzling nature of the disappearance, and the sheer sensation of it all, the human core of the story so often got forgotten. Everyone talked about what happened, while they never really discussed the truth of who it had happened to – aside from, of course, the lurid details that sold papers and boosted TV ratings. Yes, the Brindleys were tabloid-baiting in their lifestyle, but they were a family of four. Parents and two children. And the same fate befell the whole unit. The way he saw it, part of Cam's duty was to bring them home. To get these four poor people out of this unmarked sunken grave, to a proper burial. But seeing it was never going to be easy.

The adults, yeah, that would be fine. He'd fished out enough bodies during his career, in various states of decomposition and dismay. But the kids? That was something he was steeling himself for. The way the bodies would be arranged would tell their own story. About the struggle and fear. About the terror of those final moments. Even Cam, with all his frontline experience, dreaded this part.

He breathed again. In and out, slow and controlled.

This was his job. He wasn't going to let them down now.

Cam took a step alongside the car, approaching from the left-hand rear side and resting an arm against it for purchase.

Its flank seemed to gleam below darkened windows.

Two more steps. The car interior became clearer, although still a dim square. Shapes began to fashion in the darkness. Headrests. Cam steadied himself but kept going, steeling himself for what he was about to see.

He arrived at the rear passenger window, fogged with grime. He tapped on the glass and some pieces dislodged and swirled away to reveal more of the interior beyond. He brought his torch up, took a deep breath, and wiped the glass clear.

In the swirling cone of torchlight, the once-plush interior of the car was revealed in all its glory.

And it was empty.

Nothing, and nobody, was on those rear seats. No children.

Maybe, he quickly reasoned, they'd been thrown forward with the impact.

Cam angled the torch at the front seats … but there were no shapes beyond the headrests either.

He stepped to the front door and swept it clear, no fear this time, the urgency of his confusion beating back any concerns. The torch revealed the same result.

No bodies.

Where were the Brindleys?

7

They had to be here – they hadn't been seen, not one sighting of any of them, for decades. Not since the night the car went missing.

Yet now he had the car. And the family was nowhere to be found. Dread and horror trembled in his stomach.

The boot. His eyes swung to it behind his dive mask.

Were all four bodies in there? Lock a family in the boot of a car, slide it into the water? That would be some cold, old-school Mafia shit.

Cam went to the back and examined the boot's keyhole. He pressed it in, wondering if that was the release mechanism, but it wouldn't budge. He checked beneath the number plate. There – the handle. He pulled it, tugged it, but nothing happened. The boot remained clamped shut.

He paused, wondering whether he should leave the car exactly as he found it. Surely, for the purposes of whatever investigation was likely to follow, he shouldn't interfere with the evidence. But the thought of that family, stuck in that boot, scratched at the walls of his skull. If they really were in there, he had to free them.

He took his folding spade from his tool belt, the one he usually used to dig for lost bits and pieces on the riverbeds not far from here and opened it up. He wedged its flat face into the space between the trunk frame and the door, right where the handle was, and pressed down as hard as he could, trying to force the locking mechanism to release.

It was solid, but he was sure there was give in there somewhere. He heaved downwards, driving his hands to the lake bed, forcing the spade's edge ever deeper into the space between the trunk door and the car … and it popped. Air, nearly forty years old, sprang for freedom around the edges of the trunk lid, the bubbles chasing each other to the surface.

The lid roiled up with it and Cam readied himself again for awful sights.

Nothing. The only things in there were a jack and a tyre iron.

He bounced back a pace like an astronaut and stood there, feet on the bottom of Hickling Broad, staring at the empty car as the mystery transformed in his mind.

The car was no longer the mystery, although he'd always been convinced that it was the key to solving the case. He'd assumed, all this time, the car had simply gone off one of those winding roads into that ever-present water, entombing all inside in the depths. Find the car, find the family. It had never occurred to him that the car and the people who were last seen in it might have been separated.

Because as Cam stared into the empty boot of the Jaguar, the overarching question remained, now looming larger than ever.

Where on earth were the Brindley family?

All he'd taken for granted about the Brindley case had been in error. The realisation rendered Cam with a feeling of impotent loss. He hadn't failed, he reminded himself.

He'd set out to find the car, and he'd done that, but the mission had taken a turn and was abruptly only half done.

And the implications were terrible.

Because if Freddie Brindley had lost control of the car in an accident – an accident from which his family had miraculously escaped – there would have been no reason for them not to have sought help. On the other hand, if the Brindley family had simply split town in a puff of smoke as so many commentators assumed, they would have taken the car with them. Why leave it behind? Why *hide* it?

Loitering in the background of the mystery, right since the family had been declared missing, was the chance that foul play might have played a part. But to see that possibility pulled so sharply into focus caused Cam's stomach to lurch.

Now, all he was left with were more questions, and no answers came lifting from the silt beneath him.

Lifting his feet carefully, he swam around the vehicle, taking it in at all angles, looking for any hints at what might have happened before it slid into the water. His iPhone was in a waterproof lanyard around his neck, and he filmed the occasion for posterity. But as he did so, his delight at the find waned further.

Satisfied he'd had enough of his own time with the find before the inevitable chaos ensued, he swam to the rear of the vehicle. Using a screwdriver, he unbolted the number plate from the back bumper and held it in front of him. Nobody could deny what it meant, despite how unsatisfactory it felt in the moment.

But it was true. He'd done it. He'd found the car.

Taking a quick compass reading, he swam back to the bank, following the rising floor alongside the fossilised wood and sparse weeds, until he could stand. He spat out his regulator, tore off his mask, then turned and looked back at the water. There, bobbing along in innocence, was his orange buoy.

It was time to call it in.

Cam ran back to the car, as quick as his tank would allow him. Nala was bouncing up and down excitedly in the front window. He threw open the rear door and, paying no heed to caution now, dumped the tank with a clang.

'We've got it, little one,' he said to Nala while he took his phone out of the waterproof housing and dialled the number he had saved. 'We've only gone and found it.'

'Hello?' said a brisk voice on the other end of the line. 'Norfolk CID?' The regional accent was loud and clear in even this short exchange.

'Rogers?' Cam said breathlessly.

'Yeah?' The voice carried confusion now, and a hint of irritation.

'DS Claire Rogers?'

'Speaking.'

Cam tried to settle his gasps. 'It's Cam Killick here. The diver.'

'Cam… Oh for god's sake, I knew humouring you was a mistake.' The exasperation in the voice was clear.

'Are you at a computer terminal?'

'Yes, but I'm not looking up any case files for you. I've told you about this before, it's not—'

'I just want you to run a number plate,' Cam interrupted.

'You call me up out of the blue to get info from our databases? Is that what you're playing at, Killick?'

'No, it's not like that, just… Please will you run the plate.' He didn't want to tell her he'd found the car just yet. He'd had enough ridicule. He didn't want to reveal his hand without offering the proof first.

Cam could hear the distant click and tap of keys. 'I must be stupid,' Rogers said in self-admonishment. 'Go on.'

Cam held the plate up, its yellow almost burning in its brightness. 'G.'

'G, OK.'

'4, 7, 2, RSM.' Cam stated, trying to keep his voice from betraying his rejuvenated excitement. Bodies or no bodies, this was still one hell of a big deal. 'Romeo, Sierra, Major.'

'G472 RSM,' Rogers repeated – before her voice took a grave tone. 'No. No, you're joking.'

'Just … see what comes up.'

'This isn't a prank, Killick? If this is a joke, I'll drive one of those air tanks of yours where the sun doesn't shine, do you hear me?'

'Has it come up yet?'

Silence.

'Rogers?'

'You swear you're not messing around?' she replied, breathless herself now.

'I swear it. I'm holding the damn plate in my hand right now. I can show you where it is.' This is the part, he thought, where he should mention that the car was empty, and that the Brindleys themselves were still in the wind. Some snagged crease in his consciousness held him back, however.

'Stay where you are. Give me an address.'

He looked around at the swaying trees and lapping water. There wasn't a building or even a road for miles.

'It'll have to be coordinates,' he said with a smile.

8

Detective Sergeant Claire Rogers left the windows down on her black Audi estate, so she could follow the sound of sirens. They swirled everywhere, above and through the trees that reached over the roof of the car, as the emergency services converged on Hickling Broad and tried to find somewhere to park. Every now and then, the scratch of pointed wood on metal tore over the two-tone chorus and she winced at each one. This better be right, or she'd bill Killick for the damage to her paintwork. She might just bill him anyway, regardless of the outcome, for the cheek of all this.

She glanced at her phone in its cradle on the dash, the green map shorn of any road markings. The blocky shapes of the navigation app suggested that this area hadn't been reevaluated in some time, and it looked like she was simply ploughing offroad through a field. The only thing breaking the green was a block of blue on the left, denoting the roughest outline of Hickling Broad, and the red dot at the top which showed her destination – and Cam Killick's location.

Cam bloody Killick.

She shook her head. She was by now so jaded that cynicism was not just a way of dealing with things, but a character quirk so embedded it had become a central psychological pillar. And yet. She couldn't stop herself from feeling hopeful here. This case, with its individual details, quirks and parameters, was important to her – it was a core reason she'd joined the police in the first place.

Killick couldn't have found it, could he? She'd spent a lifetime wondering about this car, surely this outsider couldn't just swan in and, quite literally, drag it up from history?

The trees began to part, the branches offering the car easy passage at last, and as she saw him and his vehicle, standing in a sudden clearing on the track, she realised with a flushing tingle along her forearms that she was seconds from finding out.

The bloody diver was holding a bread roll the size of a Saxon shield, and was dressed in one of those massive, towelled poncho things she'd seen the Chelsea-tractor-driving school mums wear when they went dog-walking, as if rather than picking up their pedigree Chihuahua's crap-nuggets, they'd been out for a casual surf. Rogers pulled up behind his van, which looked far too smart and well, *nice,* for an outlier like Killick.

She stopped the engine and stepped out, instantly earning her brand-new service station wellies their first streaks of mud. She was careful to step slowly, so as not to flick mud up her black peacoat. She'd have gone home for her own wellies and more appropriate clothing, but if Killick had found what he promised he had, this place would become a circus in a heartbeat, and she wanted to be here from the beginning to stop that from happening.

'You couldn't have found this anywhere more hospitable, could you, Killick?' Rogers said as she walked carefully across the mud.

Killick gave a small smile. 'Cold cases aren't always the most considerate when it comes to location, ma'am.'

Rogers looked at him with narrowed eyes. 'Don't get full of yourself, Killick – let's see what you've got first. And if you're going to go all wanky and formal, it's detective sergeant.'

With a facial expression akin to an abruptly smacked arse, Killick meekly handed her the number plate. She made a small show of putting on a pair of latex gloves, a little reminder that Killick should have done the same.

She looked at the long strip of plastic from all angles, and found she couldn't stop her heart from thumping faster.

'It's a number plate,' he said.

Rogers narrowed her eyes again. 'I'd worked that out, thanks.' She refused to give anything away. This guy was a bloody busybody nuisance after all, crusading about the underwater environs putting himself and presumably others at risk. Her colleagues in uniform had had to have a word with him about it before. The last thing she should be doing is encouraging him, but the excitement…

If he had found what he said he had…

Killick carried on: 'It's a rear one. A rear … number plate.'

Rogers wilted his wittering with a single unimpressed look.

She flipped it over, scrutinised the back, and flicked her eyes at him. 'It appears I have a real MENSA student on my hands here.'

Killick's hands flopped to his sides, and in his oversized dryrobe he looked like a kid dragged in front of the headmistress.

'You got this out there, did you?' Rogers asked, nodding at the expanse of calm water. 'Where that orange thing is?'

Killick nodded. 'Yep. It's down there. Looks good considering.'

Rogers looked alternately between the plate and the bobbing buoy.

'Oh,' Killick said, pulling his hand back up via the pocket of his dryrobe. 'I've got this.'

He held out his phone and scrolled to a video. He pressed play and around them, the sirens seemed to grow quieter while the footage rolled. When the screen showed the front of the sunk Jaguar in all its glory, Rogers blew out a breath. 'My god,' she murmured, her own pretences withering. 'And ... there doesn't look to be anyone in it? No bodies?'

Killick sighed and nodded. 'Save for the, you know, natural wear and tear of decades underwater, it looks like it came straight out of a showroom, into the drink. But if it's the Brindleys you're talking about, then there was no sign of them.'

'No blood, clothing?'

'Not that I could see. And I confess now, I popped the boot to look in there too, but there was nothing. It would all be perfect, except I had to force it.'

Rogers looked away from the screen as the video finished, a frown creasing her brow, her eyes distant. The lack of bodies was not just troubling but heartbreaking, and going from the thrill of the mystery's supposed solving to a whole new raft of difficult questions, was hard to take. She used her trusty cynicism as a foothold and hauled herself back into the moment. 'Thanks for letting me know. I'm sure the SOCO teams will be relieved to know why it looks like the car has been broken into at six metres deep.'

Killick reddened as an ambulance came up the track behind them. It pulled up too abruptly with a squirt of mud. Rogers winced – last thing they needed was a bloody ambulance getting stuck. Two paramedics jumped out, their green scrubs spattered with mud within a few steps. The driver, a woman who walked like she was on the boiling sand of a Mediterranean beach, hopped over and said: 'Car in the water? That right?'

Rogers walked forward and in doing so, took control of the scene. This was firmly a police matter now, all earlier questions on whether this might be a wild goose chase were suddenly winging away into the far distance. 'That's right. No bodies we're aware of, but hang tight. The dive team are on their way.' She turned to Killick. 'A real dive team, with authority. No offence.'

'None taken,' he replied, but his abrupt loss of eye contact suggested some might have been.

'But best to hang on for a while in case someone turns up,' she said to the ambulance driver. 'That OK?'

'We can give it an hour I'm sure,' she replied.

'We'll take it.'

'In an hour, that thing might be sunk,' Killick said. Rogers glanced at him, then at the ambulance. He was right, but she'd be damned if she was going to admit it.

'Go and wait on the road,' she shouted to the driver, who turned and nodded.

Rogers turned back to Killick and fixed him with a steady eye. A breeze caught her fringe, but with both hands still holding the number plate, she shook her head vigorously to shift it anywhere that wasn't in her eyes. After all the time it had been hidden, she couldn't bring herself to loosen her grip for a second. 'We're going to have to interview you. We can do it here or at the station. Which would you prefer?'

Killick looked down at that impossibly happy dog, who panted back up at him from a grassy spot by his right foot. 'Here if possible.'

'Fine by me. The last thing those interview rooms need is the smell of dog piss.'

Another voice drifted on the breeze. Rogers turned to look down the track, as a rumpled-looking man charged past the reversing ambulance, up to where they were stood with the vehicles. He was shouting something, but Rogers couldn't work out the words, lost as they were in his thick grey beard and the bobbing of the flat cap he wore as he shambled along. A Brillo of hair sprang out from below the headwear.

'What does Captain bloody Birdseye want?' she murmured.

Rogers saw confrontation in his approach and felt Killick shrink back against the side of his own vehicle – a strange move for an ex-military man with his accomplishments. She tossed him the number plate, which he caught with a less-than-smooth clatter of plastic and van door and stepped forward to their visitor with her arms out, palms up like a traffic cop calling for halt.

'Sir,' she shouted. '*Sir.*'

But the man wouldn't slow. His clothes were those of the rustic gentleman, taking the style of shabby chic to all new levels of authenticity. A tired, green tweed suit, red-patterned tie, brown boots taking a progressive spattering.

He stopped in front of Rogers, his face betraying a panting exasperation – but now he was here, the words wouldn't come out.

Rogers went for the epitome of patience, although a quick sigh did leak out. 'Sir,' she said with school-teacherly calm and understanding, that belied what a ball-ache such intrusion could present. 'What seems to be the problem? Are you all right?'

'You,' Birdseye gasped, 'you…'

'Sir, take a moment,' Rogers soothed, taking one step closer.

'You can't be here,' he shouted, his arms abruptly waving towards the trees around them. 'This bit here, this is private. Private land, private water.'

Rogers couldn't hide her surprise. She glanced around. There wasn't any dwelling on this side of the water, just the reeds, the bogs and the fresh air.

But the man wasn't finished. 'You can't be here. Whatever you've found, it belongs to the water.'

9

Cam looked at the man Rogers had uncharitably called Birdseye, who was now regarding him with a manic appeal for understanding Cam couldn't reach. All it did was add to Cam's own sense of shock.

'What is your name, sir?' asked Rogers, stepping forward to head off the man's approach.

'Tabernacle,' said the man, as he took his whole beard in a fist and pulled down, smoothing it out into a point. He looked from Rogers, to Cam, and back again. 'That's Johnjo Tabernacle.'

'And what makes you so sure this land is private?'

'Because I'm its custodian. Have been for years.'

Cam didn't understand. In his research of the site, only one name kept popping up, which was the Norfolk Wetland Trust. He hadn't contacted them, admittedly, because he didn't want to get wrapped in billowing red tape – they had a habit of being pains in the arse about such things. In any event if he found the car, he was sure the drama of such a discovery and what it meant would render any trespass issues a moot point.

'This is all governed by the Wetland Trust,' Cam said. 'There's no private ownership of the water.'

Tabernacle shook his head with commitment. 'No, you see, that's where you're wrong. There's a border here on the old peat track. The way in here, that's the track. This land is private, out into the water fifty metres. The Trust only have a … a what, now … yes, an easement over it.'

Whatever Cam could understand of what Tabernacle had said, it was all news to him. 'Who owns it then?' Cam asked.

'The Belvedere Estate,' Tabernacle said, calmness arriving now he knew he was being listened to. 'They have riparian rights to the water on this side of the broad, out to fifty metres.' Tabernacle did air quotes around riparian like it was both a foreign language and password all at the same time.

It only meant more terms Cam didn't understand but would look into later.

Rogers looked at Cam, and he shrugged a *beats me*. She turned back to Tabernacle. 'And you're what, the janitor?'

Tabernacle straightened his jacket and puffed his chest out. 'I've been the custodian of the Belvedere Estate for over thirty years. Getting on for forty I'd imagine now.'

Cam couldn't help but note the poignant length of time, and its relation to what he'd found in the water. For all this time since, it appeared it had been protected by some private ownership scheme.

'And you have that in writing?' asked Rogers. 'All formalised and legal? Not just a case of you keeping an eye on things for someone?'

'Of course I do,' said Tabernacle. 'So, whatever you find in the water, I'm sorry, is the rightful property of the Belvedere Estate.'

Cam was confused. Surely the last thing any sane person would do is lay proud claim to a car that had been missing for decades in mysterious circumstances.

'What do you think I found?' Cam asked.

'I couldn't give two rats' arses,' said Tabernacle, with a jutting chin. 'Don't matter. It's not yours.'

'You can keep it,' Cam said. 'But I think the authorities might have something to say about it.'

Rogers stepped between them. 'Boys, less of it. You can measure your manhoods at the station, I'll even call ahead to get a microscope ready. I need to take statements from you both, and we are going to do it there.'

'Hang on—'Tabernacle protested.

Rogers threw twin air quotes over her own head. '*Riparian* rights or no *riparian* rights. This is a crime scene, and that means access and governance moves temporarily to us. But thank you for giving us a line of enquiry, Mr Tabernacle.'

'Crime scene...' Tabernacle said, and he turned to the ambulance as if seeing it for the first time. 'Who's hurt?'

Rogers didn't answer, because her attention had been seized by the additional police cars and vans arriving up the track. Instead, she continued: 'If this area is your job and your responsibility, then we need a serious conversation about what you've got underwater here.'

'What ... what do you mean?' He switched his gaze to Cam, who remained unmoved.

What did Tabernacle know? He seemed flustered, on the back foot. As looks went, in the circumstances, it was a bad one.

'Don't go anywhere, Mr Tabernacle,' Rogers said, before beckoning over the first arriving police constables. 'Killick, I think, when the time is right, we'll have to take both conversations down to the station.'

Cam sighed, opened his van door and sat on the step, with Nala on his lap. He sipped coffee as he watched the police work, cordoning off the area, engaging in heated little meetings. Every now and then, gazes would snap to Cam, and he found it hard not to look away. He had nothing to hide – he didn't put the damn car down there – but there was a level of confused exasperation at this interloper investigating crimes. One cop, an older one, did come over and say, 'Never thought we'd see this thing again,' before ambling off. That was as grateful a comment as he got. It made him feel like he shouldn't have called it in at all.

The police dive team, when they arrived, were far more enthusiastic, and a few of them came over to shake Cam's hand. He recognised a couple from the helicopter clean-up job that had brought him down to Norfolk in the first place, and it was nice to speak to people who *got* it – the diving, the thrill of discovery, the whole damn underwater thing. They set off into the water, and Cam felt a shared excitement at what they were about to see.

He watched and waited, his appetite growing steadily, as a helicopter arrived. It was a coastguard chopper in white and red, and it cut quite the sight as it pulled in low above the water, its rotors crashing the branches back and thumping the water in pummelled ripples. A cable was lowered from a winch and into the depths. A few wordless minutes passed as Cam imagined the dive teams below the surface, busy at work securing the vehicle. After a few moments, the helicopter gradually lifted to the sky, and the cable grew taut. It picked up height despite the weight, before slowing.

There were a couple of anxious moments then, as the helicopter seemed immobilised overhead, the only give-away that life was continuing being the spinning rotors. The cable went slack again, before the helicopter forged upwards a second time, this time with added speed, and mercifully the roof of the Jaguar crested the surface.

The rest of the car began to emerge, the sun reflecting off the window glass and body work, as the Jaguar slowly ascended like a gleaming coelacanth into the sky. There was applause from the bank and the divers in the water. Cam joined in, but it was half-hearted. His thoughts were still submerged. He looked across the broad, the only person in sight not craning their necks skyward, and watched the rolling water become calm again.

This mystery, whatever it was, remained unsolved. Where was the family? What had happened to them? He looked over at Johnjo Tabernacle, who sat on a tree stump watching the car sailing across the blue, his jaw slack with wonder and surprise.

And what, he wondered, was Tabernacle hiding?

10

Cam had been asked to wait in a stuffy side room at Norwich Police Station, and sat there in a T-shirt and board shorts, his dryrobe bundled on the floor, an old cast-iron radiator behind him pumping out so much wanton heat that one would be forgiven for thinking there wasn't a national energy crisis. After he'd been offered a drink, he'd watched as Tabernacle was ushered to another interview room further along. Cam could understand why he was second in line to be questioned – the guy had been adamant that the water and all its secrets weren't anybody's to find. His story was more urgent, in a 'suddenly made yourself seem very suspicious' kind of way.

He sipped another coffee, this one as black as concentrated tar and about as tasty, as the minutes ticked over to an hour. One hour became two. He wasn't worried about Nala – she had food and water in the van. It was himself he had to monitor. So much of military service was waiting, entrenched in a zen-like state only found through front line experience. In this zone, he could somehow rest and be alert at the same time. That was then, however. Now, he had to make every effort to ensure his calm remained intact. So far so good, but he was well aware that something small, even seemingly inconsequential, could trigger him. So he focused on small comforts, the thickness of the carpet, the warm drink and the total lack of sound, to keep his PTSD at bay. Bolstered by breathing exercises, and plenty of them.

He had been diagnosed at a military hospital in Chad, where he had been picking up extra work after he'd left the SBS. When duty and tours were over, so many soldiers were left with an impossible quandary: a lethal skill set but no place in society back in the country they had defended. Slipping back into normal life was something he'd found impossible, and he'd ended up working for a maritime security company who offered jobs to those with his particular skill set. In this instance, defending certain areas of the African coast from pirates. It was on a contract job when his world, and it felt like his very brain too, fractured, and the cost of his service was laid bare.

A third hour flirted with becoming four. Many would fiddle with their phones, but Cam didn't. He was finding comfort in the blankness of the state he'd found himself, and every now and then, danced towards the questions that hung over him.

How did a whole family just disappear?

He daydreamed about the possibilities. Had the Brindleys been fished out by water-bound grave robbers? Was there another missing Jag, identical to the first, buried somewhere else? Were the bodies in there? Had they faked their own deaths?

As the hours since the empty car's discovery rolled by, and Cam's subconscious did its job in the background, one certainty was barging front and centre.

Foul play.

The disappearance of the Brindley family, in Cam's mind at least, could surely no longer be viewed as an accident or misadventure.

Abruptly, Rogers entered with a man in plain clothes. She carried a thick file and a weary air. 'Sorry, Killick, but if you're going to crack open the county's biggest cold case, you have to appreciate that there's quite a bit of admin to wade through.'

Cam didn't move, just watched her drop into the chair opposite with a creak that could have been the tired plastic of the furniture, or Rogers' spine itself. 'It's all right,' he said, all ten fingers resting on the long-empty polystyrene coffee cup, as if he was about to enquire about the possibility of spare change. 'Although *solve* is a stretch.'

She looked up from the file as her own fingers spread certain documents on the table. The day looked to have aged her. Gone was the spiky lustre of earlier – now an exhausted concern sat in its place. She smiled tightly, glanced at the plainclothes officer, then carried on like he hadn't said anything. 'As I'm sure you can imagine, Mr Tabernacle was a priority. No offence.'

'None taken.'

She sighed and looked down at the papers. Cam looked too. Maps, and a couple of legal documents with large lettering in the top corner. TR3, TR4, they read. Land Registry papers. They looked ancient. 'What did he say?' Cam asked. He knew he was chancing his arm. The man in the corner cleared his throat, and Rogers blinked slowly.

'Forgive me, this is Detective Constable Rylance, who will be sitting in with me while we have an informal natter. That's what this is, by the way. You're not under caution, we just naturally have to get to the bottom of how you came to find that vehicle and the chain of events leading up to it. I want to make sure that, for transparency's sake, another detective was present and aware of our discussion, rather than just you and me – like all our dealings have been up to now. Of course, if you want legal representation, we can sort that out for you.'

'No, it's fine. Absolutely nothing to hide,' Cam said, glancing at the man. He had his arms folded over a baby-blue jumper, dark chinos over brown brogues. A lanyard hung around his neck, his jaw was set and free from stubble and his dark hair was cropped short. His eyes never left Cam. He could well be the most boring-looking man Cam had ever seen, but that didn't stop him from looking at Cam with unhidden suspicion. 'But you know that already.'

'I believe I do, but we still have to go about things properly,' Rogers said, pulling another piece of paper from the file and resting it on top of the short stack. She hit a button on the audio unit at the end of the table, and introduced all three present, adding that Killick had waived his right to representation. With the formalities out of the way, she wasted no time. 'For the benefit of completionism and transparency, let's get it all out there. You called me directly when you found the missing vehicle, correct?'

'Correct.'

'And for the benefit of the tape, how did we first meet?'

'At the station, here, two years ago, where we are now. I'd been asked to come in for a similar chat.'

'And why was that?'

'You know why—'

Rogers pointed at the machine on the table, the digital numbers still rolling by on its face. 'Again, for the benefit of the tape.'

'It was another occasion where I hadn't been arrested, but needed to explain what I'd been doing.'

'Which was?'

'Diving somewhere I shouldn't.'

'Where?'

'Cockshot Dyke. It's private, and a member of the public had called it in.'

'You'd been trespassing?'

'Yes, but I didn't know it was private. One of those places you can get to, but there's no signs saying it's not public. Kind of like today.'

'And what were you doing there?'

'Trying to find the missing Brindleys.'

'And you were dismissed—'

'As a complete wacko.'

Rogers offered that tight smile again. 'You had heard that tiny quote I gave that podcast a few years ago, and that's why you latched on to me, correct? Because you asked for me during interview.'

'The *Norfolk Unexplained* crew said you were in charge of old cases in Norwich CID, and you came on and confirmed there'd been no new leads in a number of years.'

'Aside from wackos ringing me up.' She smiled at him with what looked like actual admiration – maybe because it was now obvious that Cam Killick had been on the right track all along. She was thawing to him, and Cam was relieved at the thought of being believed at last.

'You seemed to care about the case. I wanted someone in the police to know what I was doing in case I got lucky and found the car.'

Rogers still smiled. 'And you liked the idea of a little official, off-the-record info if you could get it. Does that about sum it up?'

Cam reddened while Rogers turned to Rylance. 'Don't worry, DC Rylance, I gave him nothing. But it does answer the question as to how we know each other. Cam here, once we'd established that he was actively looking for the Brindleys, asked me what we knew. I said we didn't know anything, but I asked him to keep me in the loop of his activities. Gave him the number to the CID offices. Turns out he wasn't a crackpot after all.'

Rogers turned back to Cam but lowered her eyes to study the paper on the desk. 'Your records are pretty interesting.' She traced a line of text on the paper. 'Care to tell me what you were doing in Mozambique in 2004? Helmand province in 2007? Rhode Island in 2012?' There was a lilt of humour in her voice.

'I've signed the Official Secrets Act,' Cam said. 'I'm afraid that's a no.' So much of Cam's service was covered under this wide umbrella. Mute ghosts from his past that had to be left there, and yet he carried the spectres of those secrets with him every waking hour – and in many of the sleeping ones too.

'Thought as much,' Rogers said. 'Black lines through entries on a military record often tell more of a story than words ever could. Nevertheless, what I can see is a glowing career of service followed by a sad story I read all too often. Veterans who end up lost.'

Cam felt a surge of indignation at Rogers' bullseye, but her eyes carried real sympathy. 'Lots of us end up that way,' he said quietly.

'Nevertheless. You've got medals. I've heard of some but the Conspicuous Gallantry Cross? What's that for?'

'Things that don't matter anymore.'

'I understand. Along with the medals, you brought home post-traumatic stress disorder, insomnia, depression, anxiety. A hell of a trade-off.'

'If I'd have known what was coming, detective sergeant, I would never have signed up.'

Rogers blew hair out of her eyes, still examining the paper in front of her. 'How did you find yourself retiring in the Norfolk Broads?'

'I'm not retired.'

Rogers held a hand up. 'Forgive me. When did you find yourself *settling* in the Norfolk Broads?'

'It was about three years ago. I'd come to the area as part of a dive team engaged in the wreckage recovery of a helicopter from the Bure.'

'Ah yes, the one that went down outside the pub.'

'The Penny Black, right,' Cam said. He placed the cup he'd been nursing on the edge of the table. 'I'd enjoyed the dive. Found myself liking it here.'

'And you've always been a diver?'

'It was a specialism I chose to pursue in the SBS. Always loved the water, right back to being a kid. When I found out I could be a soldier in the water, it was an easy route to pick. There were a lot of practical skills that you could develop too. I liked that aspect of it.' He didn't mention that now, being underwater was one of the only mental crutches that he felt kept him sane.

'And there's a lot of water around here too, isn't there?' Rogers said. 'Had you ever been to Norfolk before?'

'Only as a kid, during the school holidays, I think. Family boat trip and all that.'

'And you decided to make a home down here?' Rogers now looked up at him, her face disarmingly encouraging. It was an interview tactic Cam was familiar with – but again, considering he had nothing to hide, he found it easy to go along with.

'When I was diagnosed with the full works and pensioned out, I found I had enough saved from that and security work to make a base here. I like the water, and the quiet pace of life suits me.'

'And you started working for yourself?'

'Yes. I can't just sit around doing nothing, and, as you said, the area is full of water. It makes sense to have a diver around.' Cam was listed online and in local business directories as a call out diver, retrieving things lost to the region's depths for a small fee. Phones and boat engines were the norm, but every now and then, he got something a touch more interesting like heirlooms or blockages. The rest of the time, he went hunting for side projects and was mapping out an understanding of the area that most people would never see. A hidden side, with a geography, contours and layout all its own.

'And you're busy?'

'It's very seasonal, like most things round here. But I don't mind.'

'And when did you first start looking for the Brindleys?'

Cam thought back to when he first heard the story, listening to the *Norfolk Unexplained* podcast in the van. It was the thirty-fifth anniversary of the mystery, a few years back, and there had been another appeal for information, although any monetary rewards had long since evaporated. A pat on the back and a snap in the *Eastern Daily Gazette* was the only reward these days, although less than that was enough for Cam. The story had caught his attention, held it granite-tight, and his search for the missing vehicle had become an obsession.

He'd started off thinking of the kids. Young kids, late at night, leaving a party. Surely, they had to be heading home.

So, Cam had immediately thought about the straight, as-the-crow-flies line between where the Brindleys left the party on the night they disappeared and their home. He'd seen just how much water they'd had to drive alongside or over, criss-crossing and snaking for miles. Cam became convinced that the water had claimed them, one way or another. And so, he'd pored over Ordnance Survey maps, broken out of his comfort zone to chat to as many local boatmen as he could, and narrowed down on the location. 'Three years ago.'

'What was it? What was it about this case that made you need to work it out?'

He opened his mouth to explain about the temptation of the water, but another answer came to him with an abruptness that forced all others out of his head. 'The family angle. The kids. The fact it was *all* of them. Families don't just vanish like that.'

Rogers smiled softly. 'I think it was a similar thing for me too.'

Cam nodded once.

'So, tell me how you narrowed it down to this spot,' Rogers said. 'Because this is needle in a haystack stuff, and nobody before has managed it. We searched all over the place at the time. Never found anything to suggest they'd gone into the water. No evidence anywhere that a car had gone off the road at all.'

Cam didn't think of it as nigh-on impossible. For him, it had been a case of twinning a methodical approach with trial and error. 'I drew a line between Norwich, where they left, and Thrigby, where they were headed. Then I went to the library a lot. Looked at any old maps I could find, both road and water. I drew my own maps from what I learned – like where roads and tracks used to be, where they aren't any more. Where bodies of water had changed in the years since. I made notes of conditions from meteorological records and eventually managed to get a complete picture of what this whole area must have looked and felt like on 7 November 1987 – both above water and below it.'

Rogers was rapt. 'With the advancements and availability of technology, even to the layperson – no offence – that probably *has* managed to eclipse what efforts we were able to go to at the time.'

'It was just a question of being methodical,' Cam said. 'Once I'd done that, I started looking at places that became less and less accessible in the intervening years. Places that were quiet, where there was protection.'

Rogers caught up quick. 'A wetland reserve.'

'Exactly. No boats are allowed on Hickling Broad to help preserve it. If the car had gone down on one of the main rivers, with boats passing over it and fishermen constantly tossing their lines in around it, it would have been found very quickly.'

'Those rivers are not that deep either. It wouldn't have stayed hidden for long.'

Cam nodded. 'So I'd narrowed it down to fifteen possible spots where a car could hide for thirty years undetected. Obviously there'd be so many more once you got out there, but these fifteen were roughly on the line between Norwich and Thrigby, on the route they were travelling, and were in areas where there had been major changes in the ecology and landscape. In this instance, I'd noticed an old border track on one of the OS maps for the peat bog workers. Forty years ago, it would still have been in passable condition for a car, but only by those who knew the area well. Now? Well, you saw it. It's a mess, and now it's not even on any maps. The track passes very close to the water – a huge body of water that recreation is prohibited on.'

'You make it sound simple.'

Cam lowered his gaze to the tabletop. 'Obviously, but with nobody actually being in the car, it's anything but.'

It was like he'd switched on a spotlight to reveal the elephant in the room. The fact that no matter how potent this buzz of discovery was, the actual root mystery hadn't been solved. Rylance unfolded then refolded his arms, stretched his brogues out in front of him. Cam thought he was going to speak, but it was Rogers who continued.

'When you were doing all this digging,' she said, swirling her hand in front of her like she was whisking a bowl of cake mix, 'did anyone come forward who gave you a golden tip? Anyone who had information that was too good to be true?'

Cam looked from Rylance to Rogers, caught by the change in direction. 'No. Nobody. I haven't told anyone what I've been doing, except for you when I rang Norfolk CID that time. I'm not … very sociable. And telling people you're trying to crack a forty-year cold case, it … well, when I've done that before I've been ridiculed.'

Rogers smiled with pinched lips. 'I imagine you'd be correct. So, Killick, there's nothing else you want to tell us about this? Nothing that you think might be suspicious if we found out about later?'

Cam thought, trying to ignore the searching gazes of the two detectives opposite him, trying to cut out the unfriendly buzz at the back of his skull. 'There's nothing. Except I'm sorry that it appears I was trespassing. At no point in my research did it come up that the land was owned, not once. I mean, I'm guessing I shouldn't have been on the wetland reserve. And diving alone, without telling anyone where I was going. That too.'

Rogers seemed to contemplate his short string of indis-
cretions with a cocked head. She then turned to Rylance,
who made no gesture at all. He barely blinked.

'OK,' Rogers said, turning back. 'Don't go far. We'll
most likely need to talk again. I think we'll need to see
some of this research of yours.'

Cam felt itchy pulses down his arms and fought the
urge to scratch. 'Of course,' he managed to say. But it was
all feeling a bit close and claustrophobic. That was how
quickly his mind could change, the symptoms of his anxiety appearing unannounced like a drunk uncle crashing a
birthday party. Tiny things set him off. Here it was just the
way Rogers had asked if he had anything to tell them. It
made him want to confess to things he had no knowledge
of.

But this time it wasn't just anxiety setting him on edge:
it was urgent questions.

Cam found, very simply, that he couldn't help himself.
'Why was the police investigation back then so short?' he
asked abruptly.

The question had Rylance on his feet, without so much
as looking at Cam, and he reached across to turn off the
recording device. Rogers opened her mouth to speak, but
Cam beat her to it.

'Four people have gone missing, they have to be somewhere. I mean no disrespect and it'll have happened before
both your times, but … the police couldn't have looked
very far, could they?'

'I can't speak for our predecessors,' Rogers said, placatingly. 'But sometimes things get missed.'

Cam felt something off about Rogers, as she looked
quickly away. Like there was more she could say but
wouldn't. He switched to look at Rylance, now pausing at

the door, and his eyes narrowing with a sudden mistrust. Rylance just stared at him with a non-committal gaze. What weren't they telling him? Where was the urgency now?

'Listen, Cam. Don't go diving in private waters again,' Rogers said, standing. 'And keep your phone nearby.'

Cam was ushered out of the interview room, shrugging on his dryrobe as he went. Sweat started to pop below his hairline. He practically leapt through the front door of the station, out into the cool press of the early evening air. He breathed, once, twice, and began to feel the tension ebb from his muscles.

'Sir,' someone said from behind him. 'Sir?'

Cam span around, and into the amber glow of the station streetlamp emerged a tall man with wild hair unsuccessfully jammed into a woollen flat cap. The tweed suit was still intact, although he'd unbuttoned it. *Johnjo Tabernacle.*

'Yes,' Cam said, feeling the burn of anxiety hit his arms and legs again.

'I'm sorry about what happened before…' Tabernacle took off his flat cap, and his hair seemed to make a break for the night sky. 'I was just a bit… Listen, do you fancy a pint?'

Cam's body and mind wanted nothing but rest. It was approaching time for another bout of medication and the idea of a social setting with other people present, people he didn't even know, made his stomach hurt.

But. By finding the car, but not finding the family, he hadn't completed his objective. The Brindley mission remained unfinished.

'Go on then,' he said. 'But we'll need to go somewhere dog-friendly.'

11

The atmosphere in Ye Olde Saddlery was low-lit and fire-crackled, though somehow to Cam the cosiness lent no warmth. Something to do with the old stone walls and the building's memories of frozen winters gone by, despite the respective advents of central heating and electricity. There was heat though, Cam noticed. Heat from the various nosy gazes that followed him as he and Nala went inside.

Tabernacle walked ahead, pointing into the depths of the building, his outstretched arm almost grazing the low ceiling's jutting dark beams. 'Let's pop back there,' he said conspiratorially. The three walked to a stone cove at the back, hewn out of ragged brick like the rest of the place – Nala giving every drinker the once-over as she ambled past. They sat on upended barrels, their top surfaces clad in tired felt, a cloudy golden pint in front of Tabernacle, a bitter lemon in front of Cam that he cradled like a life preserver.

'Sorry for holding you up,' Tabernacle said, his hands hovering as if he didn't know where to put them. 'Thanks for coming for a beer with a daft old man.'

Cam was desperate for a backrest, and his body slouched in protest. 'No probs,' he said. Nala went to Tabernacle and circled for attention, and he obliged by scratching her ears.

'I reckon I made a bit of a berk of myself out there today,' the older man said, his Norfolk accent suddenly much stronger now he was in the dark corners of a homely pub, as if he'd allowed it to be untethered. 'Tell you the truth, it's the first time I've ever had to defend that land in all the years I been keeping an eye on it. Think I got a little bit ahead of myself.'

'I had no idea anybody actually owned it. I'd have got permission to dive if I knew.' Cam wasn't sure that last part was true, but he liked to think it might be.

Tabernacle waved him off. 'Bah, it's not common knowledge. I don't even think Belvedere knows they own it anymore. They've never done anything with it. I never thought I'd be called into action, not in my lifetime.'

'How did you find out about it? That we were there today, I mean,' Cam asked.

'I live on the other side of the water, on the edge of Hickling village. I saw the whirlybird, then saw you lot in the binoculars. The blue lights, the van, the ambulance, so I drove straight round.'

'So … what's the story? With the ownership?'

Tabernacle's lip was frosted with ale froth. 'Not much to tell really. It was a long old while ago. The Belvedere Estate is the fancy name of some investment company — it's just a kind of an entity, I think, that owns land. And property and stuff like that. And people do get funny about property.'

Cam got to thinking. Buying land for investments, he could understand. Same with property. But holding onto a marshy bogland for decades? It made no sense to him, practical or financial. 'Why that land in particular? And why with those water rights too?'

Tabernacle looked more comfortable with this line of conversation, like the history of the region was second nature to him, tucked tight inside his wardrobe beside his tweed. 'The marshes are rich in peat. There's always been historical value in that, whether it be for heating in the past, or in the farming and gardening trades. And who knows what could be found under there—' Tabernacle stopped abruptly and put a palm up. 'I don't mean with what was found today, don't get me wrong. Heaven forbid. I mean like natural gas, things like that. Maybe an archae-ological anomaly of some kind. There's lots of old history in the area. Romans, Vikings, you name it. You own a bit of land, you own what's in it – whether that's treasure, or, you know, something less appealing.'

Cam could see why that first part might be attractive to an investor or owner. 'And where do the Brindleys fit in?'

'As far as I know, they don't.' Tabernacle looked befud-dled. 'Just the most awful of happenstance, is all I can imagine. The whole family disappearing like that. Gives me a stomach ache just thinking about it.'

'What do you think happened to them?' He watched Tabernacle carefully as he mulled it over.

'I have no clue, whatsoever,' the older man said. 'Until today, those poor people and the car were lost to every-thing and everybody, but always together in that sense. I don't suppose it crossed anybody's mind that they might be in separate resting places. Until you came along.' He flexed bushy eyebrows at Cam over the rim of his pint.

Cam felt again like he shouldn't have disturbed the car, nor the Brindleys' apparent legacy. Dredging things up again, quite literally, had created more questions than answers.

'Ah,' said Tabernacle, as his eyes wandered off to a spot somewhere behind Cam. They were abruptly glowing with warmth.

Cam couldn't help but turn around to see a woman, fortyish, in a dark blue fleece and work trousers, each emblazoned with the word 'Roys'. She had dyed, blindingly pink hair, with dark eye make-up and three rings in her left nostril. Cam felt heat rise up his arms in an immediate wave. He wasn't prepared for company – let alone of the female variety.

Nala, however, had no such trouble, hopping up with a wagging tail already set on high speed. 'Oh, I'd have come sooner if I'd known there was a doggo about,' said the woman, lowering to her knees to squeeze Nala tight. Something about her smile gave Cam warmth on his chest, a near-dizzying flush that darted up his neck. His left hand gripped the table as she walked over, and he forced himself to breathe.

In for a count of three.

Hold for five.

Out for eight.

He tried to hide that he was on the cusp of a full panic attack. It was amazing how quickly these things wandered out of nothingness to claim him – in this instance, the cosiest of settings being punctured by, heaven forbid, a *girl*. He cursed himself.

'Hi, Dad,' she said to Tabernacle, hugging the man tightly. Tabernacle looked at his daughter with love that shone bright between every blink. 'Fancy another pint?'

'Sure, why not?' he said, before looking across at Cam. Cam simply shook his head in two urgent jabs. The woman took a second too long to regard him, and Cam already knew what she was thinking. *She's noticed I'm a weirdo. Yep, she's seen it.*

The self-conscious burn on his chest returned.

'I'm Jess,' she said, and it pulled him back around like a friendly voice through thick fog.

'Cam,' he said – and found himself offering a hand. It wasn't his best handshake, too limp and clammy, but she took it all the same.

'And who's this?' Jess knelt down again to give Nala another squeeze.

'Nala,' he said.

'What is she?'

'A Shorkie. Half-Yorkshire terrier, half-Shih Tzu.'

Nala was gazing up into Jess's eyes as she spoke. 'So she's a proper princess until she gets the smell of something interesting, right?'

Cam found that so dead on, it caught him by surprise. 'Yeah, that's about the sum of it.'

'You after a drink yourself, Cam?' she asked, standing.

Cam looked at Tabernacle, who shrugged apologetically. 'She's her mother's daughter. Never backward in coming forward.'

This was all too familiar for him. Too weird and unbalancing. 'No, thanks.'

'Be right back,' Jess said, and mooched off to the bar.

'My daughter Jess,' Tabernacle said. 'Works in Wroxham, at the department store there. We always have a pint when she clocks off. Sorry for the intrusion.'

Cam waved it away. 'I think I best be off.'

Tabernacle frowned and pointed at Cam's glass. 'You've barely touched your fizzy thing. I wanted to know how you found that car. And what the police are going to do about it.'

'You and me both. But there isn't much to tell. I just researched the whole region, dived it a lot, came up with a hit list and boom, there it was.' Cam felt a little bad for his brevity, but he couldn't help it. He wanted to get out. Get home to Haven Cottage, get the lights off, get some medication down him, and chill. Just … *chill*.

This whole thing was threatening to get a bit too big for him. But then again, what had he expected if he found this car? A pat on the back, mystery solved and away you go? All it had offered was more questions that nagged at him, and people who wanted more from him – something that he simply couldn't give.

Jess reappeared with two pints of whatever Tabernacle had been drinking, and a huge brown dog treat for Nala. 'Is that OK?' Jess said to Cam, taking a seat next to her father. 'I absolutely couldn't help myself.'

'It's all right. She'll love you forever now,' Cam replied. He found words and gestures kept coming out of him that he was unhappy with. He felt loose and exposed. 'Well, best be off,' he said, getting up.

'Where do you live, Mr Killick?' asked Tabernacle.

What now? thought Cam. *Please just let me go.*

But he felt Jess's eyes on him. 'A place called Haven Cottage. On the way into Neatishead.'

'And you're a diver by trade?'

Cam was further surprised to find himself replying. 'Yes, all my career. First with the armed forces, now as a sort of nutter with an air tank who'll find your lost bits and pieces.'

He saw Jess smile. *Rein it in, Cameron.*

'So you have a phone number? When you're looking after large bodies of water, a handy diver would be a good person to know.' Tabernacle looked up hopefully. 'And of course, in case anything else comes up?'

That was the last thing Cam wanted. To be reachable. But he looked from Tabernacle to Jess and found himself nodding.

'I'll take it, Dad,' Jess said. She took her phone out of her fleece pocket. 'That all right with you, Cam?'

Cam nodded with a tingle in his cheeks and recited the digits.

'Thank you,' said Tabernacle, standing to shake Cam's hand.

Jess tipped her pint up at him. 'See you, diver.'

'Bye,' Cam said weakly. His neck felt molten. 'Come on, Nala.'

Tabernacle and Jess both watched him as he turned and left, his heart thumping, pleading, for a duvet, some earplugs, and his anti-anxiety meds.

12

Even though it was only eight o'clock in the evening, Haven Cottage was completely black when Cam returned. He switched the porch lights on and kicked his boots off next to the bits of post that had been delivered earlier in the day. As he crossed the threshold, he twisted the knob on the thermostat, opting for a high heat, and both he and Nala padded the wooden boards of the living room, the comforting thrum of the central heating pipes crackling to life within the walls and floors around him.

Without turning any lights on, he went into the darkened kitchen and filled the kettle. Dropped a camomile teabag into a mug. Then went to the cabinet by the sink and took out the Tupperware in which he kept his meds.

Paroxetine. Sertraline. Fluoxetine. Venlafaxine. Seven different chalky shapes on his counter in total.

Even this was only keeping the edges of his PTSD dulled for certain periods at a time. He'd done the counselling, the group sessions, the private sessions, the yoga, the reiki, even the damn healing crystals. Nothing had worked any better than the narcotic blunting he forced down his neck every morning and evening.

Kettle boiled, he poured hot water into the mug and sat on a beanbag in the living room. Nala snuggled against its base as he popped one tablet in his mouth at a time and washed it down with sips of camomile. The routine helped. So did the dark.

He ruffled Nala's ears and she yawned in response. The only light in the room was from the moon, cascading soft blue through the windows overlooking the driveway – and the green hue of the oven clock, blinking 0.00, waiting in vain since he'd moved in to be set to the right time.

It was quiet, serene, and he felt himself correcting. Like a ship in troubled waters, the pull of unseen tides began to recede, and he found himself able to think clearly.

Tabernacle was a funny guy. Curious yes, in his overall appearance and outlook, but also in his role in the land where the Brindleys' car was found. He hadn't heard of such custodian roles before. Tabernacle certainly appeared devoted to it. Cam didn't hold any suspicion of the man, far from it. He just appeared to be set in his ways and found abruptly in a situation that went way over his head.

His daughter Jess was another issue. There was something about her that he couldn't pinpoint. She was disarmingly warm, and Cam had to concede he found her attractive. That in itself could largely have been responsible for his flushes of anxiety when he met her, the kind anyone might get when they see someone that they think on first glance, is quite something. But in Cam's case, it was amplified tenfold, not just because of his riddling with PTSD – but also because he hadn't felt such a thing in years.

Literally, *years*.

He couldn't remember the last time he'd found someone attractive, because he'd closed off all that kind of contact years ago. He couldn't even remember when he'd last had sex – all right, he could, but he wasn't going to allow himself to draw that memory back into the present.

He often wondered what it would have been like, to meet someone. At forty he could be forgiven for wondering what it would be like to settle down, have children, the whole house and a white picket fence gig. He had a home already, after all, and imagined that, despite the almost oppressive quiet at times, a family might like it here.

And there it was. *A family.*

As in, some other group of people. Not him.

He couldn't paint himself into any picture like that. He simply couldn't see how he, with his problems and requirements, could ever be of use to a partner, nor children. He only saw what a burden he would be to them – and wouldn't choose to put anybody else through it.

He knew also that this wasn't about Jess, who – he chastised himself – he'd only just met. It was about the bigger picture of what his predicament and illness had robbed him of.

No wonder his mind turned to such things in the event of meeting someone, even for just a few moments.

With a noisy creak that fractured the silence, the front door handle turned.

Cam's eyes darted towards it. Nala was on her feet, looking at the handle with the same urgency.

'Kitchen,' he said firmly, and she ran through the door at the back of the living room. He jumped up, quiet as he could, and closed it behind her with a barely audible click.

Cam was shocked, the first pulses of fear beginning to accelerate. He hadn't heard anything, no footsteps outside, no voices. He went to the door, which had a flat handle, and as he walked, it angled down again in the moonlight.

Someone was trying to get in.

He crouched by the front door, staring at the handle, straining his ears through the wood. Nothing. He felt all those combat senses heighten, all those honed tingles rush back with the prospect of an apparent threat.

It was deadly silent. He looked through the key hole, and in the dim oblong of light, he could see that the porch door was yawning open at the darkness.

He caught movement. To the right of his vision. The living room windows. The moonlight beyond the glass was interrupted by shapes inching along the side of the house. Human-sized. Not just one shadow, but three.

His stomach tightened as he watched the three figures slowly progress around the side of the house. One of them stopped and pressed tight to the glass. Cupped hands on the window around eyes which were peering inside. A man. Tall. Well-built. The other two seemed the same.

They were looking for him.

Cam's old training barged into his conscious, as the man he used to be made sudden inventory of escape options. Two exits, one front, one back. Both locked. All windows could be used as exits – but as entries as well, since they were mostly single-glazed panes. Weapons to hand amounted to whatever was in the kitchen. Knives and pans and not much else.

Get low, Cam.

He slid on his knees and watched them scour the room, signal to each other with shaking heads and pointed fingers, and continue around the side of the house.

They were looking for the back door, which opened into the utility room and kitchen. Exactly where Cam had put Nala.

Fear rose, and he set his jaw, almost clenching the panic in place. He wouldn't allow them to get to her.

He thought tactically. The average person knew so little about the SBS, but they were trained up to an almost unfathomable combat readiness. Most were Royal Marines Commandos, which Cam had been himself for twelve years. It gave him tools and knowledge the average housebreaker didn't have – like the fact that he was fully aware he had the positional advantage. He knew where they were, and they didn't know where he was. But, Cam had to concede, the weight of numbers was heavily stacked in their favour.

Cam would never make any assumptions of their ability. But in murky escapades locked in classified files in the darkest corners of the Ministry of Defence, Cam Killick had beaten worse odds than this.

He looked back to where he'd kicked off his shoes by the chair in the living room.

No. The driveway was gravel, and he could easily suck up any discomfort in exchange for quiet.

Surprise was his friend. So was the dark.

He unlocked the front door, stepped outside, and slunk into the night's ink.

13

The first thing Cam needed was a weapon. Standing on his front step, the soles of his bare feet on the cold stone, he let the night air wash over him. The dank, earthen smell of freshly turned soil came with it.

He looked at his van. There was nothing in there he could use as a weapon, except, he realised, for a flare. He kept a couple for emergencies in case he needed to signal for help on one of his ill-advised solo dives. It would do for distraction at the very least.

He crept along the drive, the mud between his toes, and checked the side of the house, adjacent to where his van was resting. No sign of the intruders. They had to be round the back – that is, if there was only the three of them.

Use the intel you've got, Cam, he instructed himself. Stay cool. Stick with what you know.

He eased open the van door, his teeth bared as he tried to move it in silence, although he couldn't help the odd squeak as the runners passed along. He didn't need to move it far – the flares were mounted on the back of the front seats for ease of access. He grabbed two and left the door ajar.

With both in the same hand, he darted tight to the wall around the house – when a soft fuzziness layered on his shoulders. It wasn't heavy, it was … friendly. Comforting.

Oh god, not now, Cam thought. His meds, the meds designed specifically to calm him down, were kicking in. The last thing he needed now were his senses blunting.

Keep moving, he thought. *Fight them.*

He needed every ounce of sharpness.

He followed the edge of the house, hopping over the empty plant pots and flower beds he'd stacked there, and reached the corner.

His hearing was beginning to feel a little hollow.

The timing of this couldn't be worse. Pumping himself full of chill-out goodies, right before a home invasion… Cam cursed his bad luck.

He poked his head slowly around the corner of the gable end and looked down at the back door – where sure enough, three men stood. One, a taller man with a black beard that accentuated his jutting lower jaw, was trying the handle. He had what looked to be angel wings spread either side of his neck in an ornate tattoo. The other two were slightly shorter, flanking the big guy on either side of the faded door frame. The nearest one looked like a squat, shaven-headed Henry VIII; the other more like an aged boy band member, an earring glinting to complete the look. All three were in jeans and dark jackets. Inside, Nala was barking, muffled beyond the door.

Cam could hear them muttering to each other. Local accents, speaking in half-hushed tones.

'It's not a big dog,' said one of the shorter two.

'It needs shutting up,' said the other.

The barking wasn't putting the intruders off.

74

'There'll be a key somewhere,' the first one said, before pulling up the battered door mat.

The big one stepped over him, and tried barging the door with a shoulder, shaking the wood panel in its frame.

It forced Cam him into action.

He pulled the tab on one of the flares, which ignited with a white-hot fizz in his hand, and threw it as hard as he could into the group of men. They had turned with the cracking split of the flare exploding to life, and Cam watched their faces change as the flare flipped end over end into them. He saw gritted teeth, wide eyes and surprised expressions as the flare hit the chest of the nearest man, whose mouth split in a scream.

Cam wasted no time in ripping the other flare to life. He charged at them, but the jarring differences in colours, the brightness of the lights in his hand and tumbling to the floor, made him feel dizzy and disorientated, and he ran lopsidedly. The unwanted visitors surged to meet him, and it felt to Cam like he was watching the whole thing from a distance.

Little King Henry launched a fist, but Cam managed to drop just enough to render it nothing more than a glancing blow. Backstreet man took aim with a shoulder charge that sailed a pointed scapula into Cam's stomach. Cam felt the impact, but the adrenaline and meds stopped the pain that should have followed, and he managed to roll with the blow, sending his assailant slipping on the mud. Cam staggered back, fighting for balance, then running off a drunken kind of instinct, jabbed Little King Henry in the cheek with the burning end of the flare. The scorched man let out a wild howl. With his left leg, Cam then stamped on the ankle of Backstreet man, brought his foot up, and stamped down again, this time on the knee.

Still clutching the flare, Cam swung it across to the big man in the middle, but his aim felt skewed, like looking through a sniper scope in a typhoon. He missed, poking wildly at the air. The big man pushed him backwards.

'You're one dead fucker,' he seethed.

Cam tried again to swing the flare across all three men – when he felt a thud on the side of his own head, and sparks popped in the corner of his vision. He heard the metallic spit of something being flicked to full extension, and just caught sight of the telescopic baton as it buried itself painfully in his gut.

It felt like a bomb had detonated, deep in his stomach. He fell to his knees and took a kick in the side of the head, which sent him sprawling face down into the dirt.

'Sneaky bastard,' said the big man, unscathed, bearing down on Cam with the baton. 'Get that dog to shut up or I'll skin it and wear it as a fucking hat.'

Nala was going ballistic on the other side of the door, barking and scratching. Cam spat blood, which looked like globs of oil in the flickering light of the downed flares. A tooth was loose, and his tongue felt like a slug lolling about in his mouth. 'Nala, quiet girl,' he croaked. He pulled himself to his knees and took a full punt to the kidneys.

'That's for my fuckin' face,' seethed Little King Henry, pawing at his injured cheek with both hands.

Backstreet man, the one with the mangled leg, tried to swing his own foot at Cam, but couldn't lift it. 'Jesus,' he hissed before dropping onto his knees again. 'You've broke my ankle.'

Everything in Cam's body hurt, but thanks to the wash of meds pumping through his system, he felt detached from it. Like it belonged to him, all that pain, but only vicariously. He felt its pointedness only through a veil.

'This was only supposed to be a chat,' said the big man, who Cam had come to think of as the leader of this particular posse. The voice was a bark which promised bite. 'But you dragged it somewhere really unnecessary.'

Cam spoke through the blood in his throat and the haze in his head. 'You tried to break into my house. I'd say *that* was pretty unnecessary.'

That earned Cam a harsh whack on the top of his arm from the baton, an impact which rattled right across his body. 'Keep your gob shut.'

Cam did as he was told. The man took the invitation to continue whatever spiel he'd come to deliver. 'Don't speak, just nod. You're the diver that lives here?'

Cam nodded. It hurt.

'I need an ambulance,' Backstreet man gasped from the darkness nearby.

'I do too,' said Little King Henry, still pawing at his burnt face.

'Shut up, you idiots,' the main man shouted.

'But my leg is fucked!'

Cam turned to look. 'It's his ligaments,' he said through tired breaths. 'Six months of physical therapy and he'll tango again.'

The main man laughed. 'You a doctor?'

No, Cam thought. But that told Cam something new. They knew very little about him. Only that he was a diver. *Good.*

'Enough mucking about,' said the main man, stooping to Cam's face. 'The Brindley car. What else did you find in it?'

His words surprised Cam. The discovery of the Brindley car hadn't been reported yet. He fought to make a connection between what seemed like a piss-poor burglary attempt and the events of the day.

'I don't understand...' Cam started, but the big man grabbed him by the cheeks and pulled his whole head up for inspection.

'Never mind the simpleton bullshit – what else was in the car?'

'Nothing, it was empty,' Cam gasped.

The man gripped Cam's cheek's so tight his nails dug into the skin. 'I want you to think very carefully before you lie to me.'

'There was no one in it,' Cam insisted, coughing.

'Nothing in the back?' the man said urgently.

Cam found his word choice odd, but mirrored it. 'Nothing.'

The man looked deep into Cam's eyes with searching intent. 'Are you sure?' His breath smelt like Frazzles, booze and menace.

'All right, now you listen. You're going to forget the whole damn lot.' The man lifted Cam's chin up again, but he could barely feel the fingers on his skin now. 'Do you understand that? Or do we need to hurt you some more?'

Cam looked at him as defiantly as he could, but on a one-to-ten pain scale, the meds' fog left him on what he was sure was a three.

'Who are you?' Cam managed to say through the blood in his mouth.

'Don't matter, does it,' said the man. 'The only thing you should be thinking about is amnesia, and how quickly you can find it.'

'You didn't answer my question.'

A boot to the guts from Little King Henry went some way in response. Cam's breath left him in full, and his teeth reflexively bit for air. The new pain in his side punched through the meds, like a giant hook had been jammed in his flank and twisted.

He felt his body make its first lurches to shut down, and his head dipped to the earth, filling his nose with the incongruously pleasant notes of petrichor. Nala seemed to sense his agony and barked in a tone he'd never heard before.

The big man stepped forward again, now with the baton raised high. 'You forget the car and leave it well alone. And if that message has somehow got confused because you've had a couple of knocks to the head, we'll remind you by burning this house to the ground with you and your dog in it. Understood?'

Cam looked up at him with flaming defiance.

'Now, sleep' – and he punched Cam so hard, Cam didn't even have time to realise it had gone dark before he was out.

September 1987

'Come on now, nearly there,' I say to the bundle of fur in front of the kitchen Aga. I put her there for warmth. 'You've done so well.'

I stare into those big eyes and give a smile I hope looks full of kindness. She looks like she's begging for something. I stroke the dog's head and look back at her, trying to send as much strength and power through to her as I can. 'Having babies is hard, isn't it!'

It is late afternoon and summer is pretty much over. Back to school tomorrow. I'm nervous about it – but I also can't wait to tell everyone about this whole litter of brand-new puppies.

I put my hand on the dog's belly and feel along its ridges. There it is. With my thumb and first finger, I pinch and open the Velcro strap. I poke my hand into the dog's fluffy guts and one at a time, pull out a litter of super cute puppies that look just like their mother.

One of them makes a squeak when I squeeze its belly – its first sound!

I put them next to their mother, thinking of all the personalities they will have, and fold shut the Velcro with a pat.

Pound Puppies are just amazing, and the new pregnant one with babies is the best thing ever. Dad got the toy for me, to say sorry for being out all the time.

I'd rather he didn't have to say sorry.

It's why I'm in the kitchen now.

I couldn't bear to hear the noise from upstairs.

Raised voices, changing from booming to hushed whispers whenever Mum and Dad remember their children can hear them. It never usually bothers them though, who hears.

I have no idea what they are shouting about today. They always seem to be upset.

The kitchen door behind me creaks, and I turn to look. It's Tommy, his Luke Skywalker haircut coming in before he does, just like always.

'Are you OK?' he says, his own face full of apologies that should be coming from people far more grown-up than him. He's eleven, four years older than me, and I'm always grateful, when he looks at me like he is now, to be his little sister.

'Yes,' I say – but just from him asking, I feel tears I don't want prickling the corner of my eyes. I push them away, quick as I can. They never change anything. 'Have they stopped?'

He turns and listens into the depths of the house. Dad recently decided to change its name to Brindley Hall. It used to be called Feather House, which was much better. Brindley Hall sounds like a museum where ghosts bang on doors in the middle of the night.

Tommy turns back and shakes his head with a tiny smile, his eyes sadder than my Pound Puppy's. 'Not yet. I think they're getting ready for another big blast.'

'OK.' Without thinking, I seem to have picked up one of the stuffed puppies and am stroking the top of its head with a thumb. Back and forth, back and forth.

Suddenly, a door slams somewhere above us. It is so hard it sets the windows rattling and I feel it right through the kitchen ceiling.

'I'll tell you when the coast is clear,' says Tommy, and he blows me a kiss. I blow him a kiss back, and he leaves with the soft click of the kitchen door.

I can feel another sorry present coming on, so I get back to stuffing the babies back into their mother's belly. The mother's drooping eyes seem to stare at me. The stuffed dog looks about as sad as I feel.

14

It was the cold that brought him round. Frigid moisture, straight through his clothes, like a mild burn on his skin.

The smell of soil came next. A smell so ancient and rooted in human history, he didn't even have to think to identify it.

Then barking. *Nala*.

He opened his eyes, to find one was glued shut with something cool and clogged. The pain that rushed in with his growing consciousness reminded him of the beating he had taken.

With one good eye, he saw the cornfield that he knew was behind his home – even though the tall stalks were now horizontal thanks to his position on the floor.

'I'm here, Nala,' he said, but his voice cracked as it left his throat. He coughed and cleared it, then pulled himself up. The ache in his side was pronounced, like a knife had been stuck in and left there for the wound to fester. Gingerly, Cam eased himself into a sitting position and took a practised inventory of his extremities.

Two legs. Two arms. He was capable of thought, so he knew he had a head, but he ran his hands through his hair to check for damage. A bit of blood came back on his fingers, but no major leakage. His torso was a wrought, ringing block of low-level agony. All internal, no open wounds.

The main issue seemed to be his eye, which he knew not to touch.

'I'm here, Nala,' he said again, reaching for the bottom step. She whined. He edged closer, past the stone paving slab of the entrance, to a dirty pottery frog that stood guard by the door, its faded bug eyes regarding him as if through cataracts. He took the ornament and flipped it over. The spare back door key sat there, as it had since the day he moved in.

Nala snuffled at the bottom of the door frame, her claws clicking on the tile of the utility room.

He opened the door while still on his knees, and as soon as it swung inwards, Nala rushed out. She was light, but excited, and the force of her approach pushed him onto his back. She pawed and licked, but after a poor attempt at hugging her, all Cam could do was lie there as she scurried around him.

He stared at the stars overhead. Crystal, they were. Constellations visible as far as his one eye could see, some with whipping nebulas loosely connecting them.

Leave the car alone.

The message was clear. But he had no idea who it was from – which would go a long way, he guessed, to explaining the message in the first place. But it was the question which came prior to the order which bothered him the most.

What else was in the car? Nothing in the back?

They knew he'd been down there and seen the Brindley car in person. And yet their question hadn't been about the family. No, Cam was sure of it. They never once mentioned the bodies.

Nothing, was the word they'd used.

They weren't interested in the possibility of bodies at all. So what *else* was supposed to be in the car?

The ringing in his head couldn't mask the stark realisation that those people, surely, knew something about what happened that fateful night forty years ago. Why else would they have come so quickly, on learning that someone had gone poking around in the past? You simply didn't come knocking out of the blue if you didn't have a vested interest.

And yet, Cam thought, none of them had looked old enough to have been similarly active in the eighties. Cam guessed the thugs were a similar age to himself, or even a touch younger. So, who were they? Who did they represent?

Somebody, it seemed, who could send three goonies out in darkness to deliver a message with violence, armed with a telescopic baton that you couldn't pick up down at the supermarket.

I don't want this, he thought, as he watched a tiny grouping of lights forge a straight-line path across the cosmic tapestry. An aeroplane, on the way somewhere nice, he imagined. All he'd set out to do was find the car – not uncork a decades-old can of worms that could come knocking at his door.

He felt Nala's attentions get closer to his face – and that eye.

'Inside,' he said. Nala moved to the door, then turned and looked at him with a cocked ear, as if to say, *well, are you coming?*

'Yeah, yeah,' Cam said as he hauled himself to his feet. Groggy didn't cover it. Seasick was more like it.

He stumbled into the utility room and closed the door behind him. He pulled his T-shirt over his head and shimmied carefully out of his joggers. Boxers too, and he groaned as he bent to put them in the washing machine.

Now fully nude and in the dark, the quiet was bringing multiple truths with it. Painful, difficult ones. The internal bruising and crushing disorientation of a concussion were obvious. Along too came the cheese grater scrape of anxiety, the needles of outside pressure puncturing the protective membrane the meds had given him.

He found the sink, ran the tap. Washed his hands as the washing machine clunked to life and started to whir obnoxiously. Above the basin was a square mirror, spattered by dried water drops he hadn't wiped. It gave his reflection an even more fractured quality than he felt inside.

His quiet bubble had been shattered. His rebuild, the very reason he was here in this house, in Norfolk, was under attack, and it lit a fire in Cam that he wasn't sure he was ready to carry. And yet, he already knew he wanted to see those men again. To try again. On a different day, under different circumstances, with a different outcome he was suddenly hell-bent on.

In the dim light, his right eye was black.

He looked at his watch, still on his wrist from the dive. It was only 9:42 p.m. He'd been out on the ground for maybe ten minutes.

The whole attack had taken barely any time at all – and certainly not enough time for an injured eye to become as blackened and congealed as Cam's appeared to be.

He reached up, and gently prodded the edge of the dark mass. He didn't feel a thing. He poked the centre – nothing again. *Jesus*, he thought, *did they gouge it out?* He pushed harder with his finger tip and something fell off his face, with a wet plop into the sink. *Oh, god…* He looked down at it, terrified, but all he saw was a blob of mud with a couple of blades of grass in it.

He looked closer at his face, leaning nearer the mirror, and breathed a sigh of relief. He pinched the edges of the blackened mass and pulled out another clod of mud. With it, his vision returned.

He smiled. The endorphins that came with the relief gave him much needed strength, as he scrubbed the mud away.

'Come on,' he said, and Nala followed as he made his way out of the utility room, through the kitchen and up the stairs, leaving every room dark as he went.

He went straight into the bathroom and sat on the edge of the tub as it filled with tepid water, going over and over the attack in his mind, the endorphin rush soon fading, the fears and tension cramming back in.

He watched the bath fill, urging it to go faster, now desperate for restorative solace.

The throbbing in his head wasn't just the physical discomfort. It was the ache of the mystery. Since finding the car, new layers were unravelling fast – and he felt a dutiful pull, despite the warning he'd been so painfully given. He had growing, pressing questions about just how rigorous the police investigation into the Brindley matter had been if, nearly forty years on, the resurrection of the topic was suddenly bringing violence with it.

Present-day Cam knew he needed to take stock and recuperate, but all-guns-blazing, past-Cam also yearned to sprint downstairs, into the car, and head off into the night to pull the Brindley mystery apart, piece by secret piece.

That is, if his aching legs would carry him. Because he simply wasn't that man anymore.

Really, he knew he should call the police. Ring the emergency services and report the attempted break in and his assault. That's what a normal person would do.

But he just couldn't face the questions. Not again, not after the day he'd already had – never mind how much his head hurt.

The bath was done, and he wasted no time. Nala took her place, curling up on the end shelf, while he took the snorkel and dropped straight in under the water.

The effect was almost immediate, and his muscles began to loosen. They were so contracted that it would take some time – but it would happen eventually. He lay on his back and forced his shoulders to ease against the porcelain of the bathtub.

And as they finally got there, his brain emptied and the quiet arrived. The last thing he thought before sleep took him was that he, Cam Killick, whether he meant to or not, had stirred things up big time.

15

Even underwater, the effects of the morning's headache were all-encompassing. It surprised Cam when he woke, considering how much being submerged usually remedied him – but then he remembered the beating, and chose to lay there for a few more moments in the cool water.

He wasn't sure if he was ready to get out.

Face the inevitable pain.

Face the music of the mysteries he'd resurrected, swirling in his subconscious with the persistence of an unwanted soundtrack.

But the longer he lay there, the more he thought he was dodging the issue, and that irked him. No marine, and no SBS boy, ever shirked duty.

He sat up, and sure enough, as the water ran off his body, the hard deep aches of the pummelling set in. Willing his eyes to open, he found that it was dawn, with the bathroom bathed in magenta from the windows.

Red sky in morning. Shepherd's warning.

Nala was curled like a C, with her head on her front paws. She watched him with regal curiosity.

'Morning,' said Cam, offering her the snorkel tube. She took it between her teeth and went to gnaw on it at the foot of his bed. It was then he noticed the colour of the bath water – a mucky, brownish pink, where all the blood and mud had fallen off him overnight. He pulled the plug, watching it all get sucked away, an unpleasant swirling reminder.

Hauling himself gently up, he left the bath to switch the shower on, opting for hot this time, and soaped himself down. In the mirror, he checked for wounds, the sun higher and brighter now. There was swelling in patches all over his face, with a few cuts in bolts of blue and purple. In his hair somewhere near the back of his head he could feel a gash. He had a flash of memory as he probed it, of the telescopic bat glinting in flare-strobe light as the thug swung at his head. He was pretty sure he had a concussion too.

It was a hospital job, even though he didn't want it to be. His rule for assessing himself for injuries was simple: *would I send someone else to hospital who had the same injuries as me?*

If the answer was yes, he made himself go.

There was no point trying to be a hero – especially not when he had all those medals somewhere that said he was one anyway. He would go.

Cam flipped open the mirror to reveal his well-stocked medicine cabinet and started taking out blister packs and arranging them on the edge of the sink, long-embedded routine guiding his movements. But then, abruptly, he stopped himself.

His head was throbbing because of the bashing it took the night before. And he firmly believed that he got himself into that predicament because he was slowed down, rendered languid by the tablets he had diligently funnelled into himself.

The tablets, while softening the edges of his anxiety and paranoia, had cost him the combat edge which could have averted what happened. Cam Killick, the soldier of a few years back, would have no doubt won, because that was simply how he'd been conditioned to see objectives. It was the winning mentality of a champion boxer. *I'm going to win — because if I even contemplate losing, the door is left ajar for doubt to creep in.* You win because you've left no room for failure — and you prepare for the situation with that same winner's mentality.

Cam looked at the blister packs, half-popped, with twists and flecks of silver foil poking out across one side of the two rows. These had helped him, no doubt. They had righted the ship when his own storms had threatened to sink it, and they'd taken the sting out of some of the heavier blows. But his current more sedentary lifestyle had hidden just how much he'd come to rely on them. And now there were people watching him, he had to keep himself sharp. He questioned whether he still needed them.

The bruises on his face told him the answer. The debilitating nature of his condition, he was aware of and prepared for. Defending himself at half-speed, he was not. These drugs simply wouldn't do right now.

Cam shelved the blister packs, and gingerly walked into the bedroom to get dressed.

16

Claire Rogers sat in bed, a cold cup of tea on the night table next to her, and an iPad propped up on her knees, the screen long ago dimmed out through inactivity. Beyond the curtains, the birds had been at it for hours, but their nuisance chirruping hadn't been the thing that robbed her of sleep. Restless, she decided to read. The book was great, but nothing was keeping her mind off the day before. Her get-up time of 6 a.m. was fast approaching and so little was her chance of sleeping, she'd switched the alarm itself off.

There was so much to do today that her legs oddly ached at the thought of staying still any longer, in some oxymoron of physiology. It was going to be a huge day, because the story was about to break. Thanks to Killick's natural proclivity for keeping himself to himself and the remoteness of the car's final resting place, it hadn't been that hard to keep the matter under wraps so far, but it was only a matter of time before it leaked, and chaos erupted. To head this off, and stay ahead of things, the chief was holding a press conference, and the world was going to find out that the Brindley car had been found.

For Rogers so much of that statement was the very problem that kept her awake.

Car.

Moreover, *just* the car.

Killick was right, and she knew it – the fact the car was empty left even more unanswered questions and secrets to find. It also meant the very question of why she'd got into policing was still far from answered.

She looked out of the window of the small townhouse in the centre of Norwich that had stretched the limits of her salary for years, at the early morning buses lined up along the road ready for another day to start proper.

When she first joined the police, people had asked her why. *Why would you want to do that, Claire?*

She usually offered the expected answers. *Oh, you know, to make a difference.* As years went by and the weight of the job dulled her hopes and jaded her intentions, the answer changed to something more akin to *Well, it's better than sitting on my arse.*

The real reason, she had told nobody. Not even her parents, who were sitting in a nursing home in North Walsham, merrily whiling away their twilight years feeding ducks and playing bingo.

There was no coincidence that she was in possession of Norfolk Constabulary's case file on the Brindleys. She'd sought it out, requested it, kept it close. All because of Tommy Brindley. The eldest child in the family. She'd been in Scouts with him. She'd babysat for the children a few times. And when they'd disappeared, without so much as a clue, it had haunted and shocked a then-teenage Claire. She'd found it unfathomable that there were no answers. Unconscionable that those children could go missing, never to be seen again, right there, where she was growing up. Back then, she'd found herself crippled by the uncertainty that lack of answers brought and felt the same feeling now. Young Claire had decided that if she couldn't find them, she'd try to make sure that such uncertainty would linger over as few families as she could. So, she'd joined the police.

When it came to the Brindley case, there'd been no progress in years until Cam bloody Killick came along and blew the whole thing wide open.

She would never give him the satisfaction of outright saying it to his face, but what Killick had done was utterly remarkable. He'd found vital evidence which forever altered a case that was almost forty years dead. In investigative terms, that kind of thing was a unicorn in stature and rarity. He had used advances in modern technology, sure, but the root of his thinking was based in logic, experience and good old-fashioned hunches. The fact that he was socially unaware of his feat made the achievement all the more impressive.

The jammy bastard. All that effort she'd put in, only for some loon with a snorkel to come along and make the biggest breakthrough the case had seen in years.

She also felt sorry for him, however, again something she'd never give him the satisfaction of knowing. Duty came at a cost to everyone who served others, and the scale of the cost varied from case to case. It just so happened that Cam Killick was paying a debt so heavy, the severity of it was clear in his every action. The poor guy was tortured, tormented.

Her mobile phone rang from the bedside table by that ruined cup of tea. She grabbed it quickly before it could wake Martin, but he still managed a sleepy grumble next to her. 'Can you get that please?'

'Sorry, my liege,' Rogers grovelled in an exaggerated voice.

Ordinarily she would've taken it outside onto the landing or perhaps into the kitchen, but thanks to Martin's twattishness, she'd have the conversation right there, thank you very much. She might even shout it. 'Rogers?' she answered, too loud. Martin huffed next to her.

'Rogers, it's Rylance here.' *That officious little toad,* thought Rogers. Rylance didn't wait for her to speak.

'We need you to come in early, please. The chief wants a debrief.'

'Debrief? I filed my reports last night, and as much as I know he enjoys the sweet tang of progress, I'm afraid not much has happened while I've been, you know, in bed.'

Remembering that Rylance was essentially a direct line to the chief, primarily thanks to just how far his nose was buried up his backside, she eased up on the sarcasm. 'Has he not seen them? He can just read them and be all caught up.'

'The debrief is not for him, it's for you.'

'What?' she sat up in bed and had now raised her voice unintentionally.

'The feeling is, with the case closed, we can finally put the whole thing to bed. The chief is clearing it.'

Rogers couldn't believe what she was hearing. 'What on earth are you talking about? You sort of need to solve the crime before you just go ahead and clear it?'

'Well, the matter is resolved, after all,' Rylance said, no understanding or empathy in his voice. Worse than that, there was no bend. 'The chief says it's closed, and he wants you to be there, for the formalities. Seven-thirty.' Ryland hung up before she could say a further word.

She sat there stunned.

'I don't believe this,' she said.

'Neither can I,' said Martin, whining as if he'd just endured the greatest inconvenience. 'You didn't even go outside.'

'Oh would you just piss off, Martin.' Rogers was raging. Her tone said it, and it persuaded Martin not to add anything further.

She got up, her head swimming with all the reasons why this case couldn't be cleared. She couldn't understand what her own force was playing at, but worse than that, it gave credibility to the points Killick had made, and her own concerns she had tried long ago to bury.

Namely, why had the police come up so short in finding them? Why had her own force achieved nothing in almost four decades?

She'd always wondered if their inability to solve the matter at the time was down to the shortcomings of the available technology and techniques … or if there had been something more willing about the shortcomings.

With the suggestion that the case was being brushed under the carpet, an uneasiness swept across her. She quickly got dressed, ready to fight for the case, and justice for the Brindleys, to stay alive.

17

The hospital visit had taken almost all morning, the waiting times in accident and emergency glacial in their turnaround. It had been a struggle to keep it together, with the hectic peaks and troughs of triage constantly provoking his senses. Cam moved from plastic seat to plastic seat regularly to reset and occupy himself with small changes of perspective. He used breathing exercises with a near-religious devotion, at one point forcing himself to stare at a wall and nothing else, until eventually he was called in.

Mercifully, his injuries were nothing worse than expected, his own self-assessment ringing true. The gash on his head was stitched up by a nurse who was more than a little heavy-handed, but before long he was discharged and on his way back to the van, and Nala, who sitting on the front seat, had snoozed her way through the whole lot.

His next port of call promised to be much more engaging.

He was going to see Rogers and eke as much as he could from her about where the Brindley case was up to – and maybe tell her about last night's visitors.

He drove to the station – and parked on a side road. It felt like weeks since Johnjo Tabernacle had poked his head out from under a streetlight and asked him whether he'd like a beer. It seemed that a blow to the head offered the same sensations as a trip in the DeLorean. He hopped up the lone front step, his gait jerky with urgency, and asked the desk sergeant for DS Rogers.

'What is it regarding?' said the man, casting a dubious glance over Cam's wounds while taking the phone off the receiver.

'Just say it's Cameron Killick – she'll know,' Cam replied, with confidence.

The desk sergeant looked at Cam nonplussed, like he'd just dropped his trousers to proudly reveal he was adorned like a squirrel and blinked slowly. 'OK, please take a seat and I'll give her a buzz.'

Cam, embarrassed, sat down. A few moments passed, during which he switched seats a few times and counted backwards from a hundred, before the door at the end of the waiting room opened and out marched Rogers. She looked tired and hassled, the case evidently taking an early toll. Rather than call him through to the interview rooms, though, she walked straight past him to the front door, and cocked her head in the direction of the daylight. *Follow me.* Cam did as bid, and as soon as they were outside, she marched off down the street at such a rate that he actually had to jog to keep up with her – which did nothing for the ache in his side.

'Never mind dragged, you look like you were forced through a hedge by a backhoe,' she said, without even glancing at him. She was on edge, constantly checking her periphery.

'Feel fairly similar. Where are we going?'

'Somewhere else,' she said.

It turned out that 'somewhere else' was a Wetherspoons pub, where cheap ale flowed and early afternoon drinkers already had most of the tables choked. It hit Cam like a wall of needles, but he gritted his teeth and breathed slowly, imagining he had an air tank on his back. Rogers ordered a glass of Sauvignon and offered Cam a drink, but he shook his head. She shrugged, and watched as a glass of off-white liquid was poured from a tap mounted on the bar.

Cam could barely contain his surprise. This wasn't the Rogers he had come to know, albeit in his extremely limited capacity. Bringing a witness to a *pub?* Drinking on the job? Her behaviour was wildly, weirdly unprofessional, her manner all kinds of *off.*

Once she had her drink, Rogers headed through the crowds and dark wood panelling to a spiral staircase offering further seating and toilets. Each step piled on Cam's discomfort, each extra second in here driving his senses bananas.

'A booth,' he said when they reached the top and another dimly lit prison of dark wood, pointing to a spare table at the back under a painting of fish playing backgammon. By the time he slumped down, he wished he'd asked for a glass of water.

Rogers seemed to notice his discomfort; at any rate her blunt facade faltered a little to reveal concern. She glugged from her glass, the large wine taking a serious dent. 'You do look like shit, you know.'

Cam breathed heavily, counted backwards again, trying to get the smallest measure of control back. 'That's what I'd come to tell you about. I had visitors last night. Three men – asked me what was in the car, then told me to leave it alone. They laboured that last point with a telescopic baton.'

Rogers looked up into his hairline, evidently taking in his injuries. 'I'd listen to them.'

'I haven't worked out where they were from yet, but—' Cam stopped in his tracks, his words on pause as they left his lips. Rogers' face was a picture of resignation. 'You're serious,' he said.

'Please, Cam,' Rogers said. There was a graveness to her tone, and melancholy in her eyes. 'Look, the official line, the one I'm *celebrating* right now, is that the case was open and shut.' Sarcasm was layered thick as she picked up the wine glass once more. 'You did a great job, you solved the whole thing. The Brindley case is closed. You're a hero, and now we all have to leave it be.'

Cam couldn't believe what he was hearing. 'What the hell do you mean? Forgive me stating the obvious, but there's still four people missing.'

She sighed and spun her wineglass slowly on the spot. 'There aren't. You found them, but decomposition had done its job – apparently. There was nothing left to find.' She could barely look at him. The penny dropped hard, Cam's stomach with it.

'You've been told to drop it. This is an order, isn't it?' Cam knew bullshit instructions when he heard them; he'd been on the receiving end often enough.

Rogers, although she still couldn't look at Cam, glared into the distance. 'What do you think Rylance was doing there yesterday? He's the chief's loyal terrier, got his eyes on the top jobs. He was there to oversee our conversation and report back.' The disdain in Rogers' words was blatant.

'But surely your bosses know that this thing is far from over? We need to find that family.'

'Yep. That's why I've decided to take our meeting in a more *liquid* direction.' She sipped another dent in the huge glass.

'You're not going along with this, surely?'

Rogers finally looked at him, her expression one of raw sadness, any pretence of bravado fully eroded. 'I have to, Cam. I don't have a choice.'

'This can't happen, Rogers. I'm not going to let it lie, those people last night—'

'Are sadly irrelevant.'

He looked at her, feeling every one of his bruises burning defiantly on his face and body. He couldn't believe what he was hearing. 'Not irrelevant to me. This is a joke. And you know it.'

Rogers didn't reply. Cam wanted to get up and march out. He'd seen this in his military career. People behind desks giving orders based on only a small portion of the information to hand. No clue, no fraction of an idea how things worked down on the ground. To say this case was closed, to Cam, was nothing short of immoral.

Who had instructed the case be closed so quickly? How could they possibly see it as that cut and dry? These new questions now sat along all the others, a host of unruly voices demanding attention like infant birds clamouring in a nest.

'You know how corrupt this conclusion sounds?' Cam said with no small amount of accusation.

Rogers' eyes finally met Cam's as she leaned forward. They were wide with pleading. 'Look. What I'm about to say can go no further than this table. I know what you've done, I know what stellar work you put into finding that car. It was a one in a million shot and you pulled it off. You're right, this whole thing deserves more.' She looked at the tabletop as if the right words could be found in the whorls of the cheap walnut wood. 'I was dragged in to see the chief today. Rylance was there, but don't get me started on him. There's a press conference later. I thought, when it was booked in yesterday, it would be to announce the true status of the case. Instead, the media is going to be briefed with this apparent resolution, wrapped in a neat, tidy bow. It's going to be chalked up as a resounding win for justice and our police force – even though everyone knows it was you that found it. The Brindley file has been closed at last. That's the official line. I protested as strongly as I could, but there's a limit to what you can do when your job is threatened.'

'They threatened to sack you?' Cam asked.

'They did. Told me that I was to leave the Brindley case well alone, that orders had come from even higher than the chief's office. We're all to move on.'

'But *why*?'

'I don't know, Cam. But I'll lose my job if I don't do as I'm told. I'm nigh on thirty years in here, on the road to a half-decent pension. I can't afford to lose that.'

'So you're taking the money.'

She pointed at him sternly. 'Hey. Don't be a dick. I...' Her gaze drifted again, unable to meet nor match the fire in Cam's. She closed up, both in words and in body language, and Cam could see there was no point trying to push the matter further. Rogers' hands had been tied. Worse than that, her superiors had closed the whole thing, rubber stamped it as a job well done.

Cam got up to go.

'You might be under orders,' he said. 'But I'm not.'

'I thought you might take that line,' Rogers said – and she was smiling so softly it might not have been there at all.

She passed a card across the table. Unmarked. A number starting with 07.

A private mobile number.

For Cam, it took a second, but it clicked.

'Don't do anything I wouldn't do,' she said.

'Yes, ma'am,' Cam said with a tight smile of his own.

He walked out of the pub, and into the street, buoyed by a small wave of encouragement. Rogers was giving him the unofficial nod to explore other avenues, and it was something a man like Cam Killick could really get his teeth into.

He decided to strike while the iron was hot, if only in his mind – and took his phone out, to uncharacteristically slide into some DMs.

18

Cam took the ring road north out of Norwich, towards Sprowston, Broadland and the very rivers that this mystery seemed mired in. He quickly found himself winding around a couple of rolling, wood-clad bends, which was quite disorientating, given that only moments before he'd been wading through the congestion and pace of the city centre itself.

He soon found where he was headed as it appeared to be the only building around, clinging to a bend like a lone barnacle on a sea serpent's gut. Cam, aware of its history, had always wanted to visit and was grateful for the excuse. It was a mock-Swiss pavilion, built in 1901 as a hunting lodge on the cusp of the wild trails of Mousehold Heath: a place to knock back a couple of winter warmers before heading out into the snow to murder a deer.

As he parked the van alongside a couple of other vehicles just off the road, he saw a neon sign in that traditional handwritten font known by boozers the world over, hanging between the first and second levels of the building. 'Rodney's', it said. It was the most jarring mish mash of styles Cam had ever seen.

He wasted no time in jogging up the short driveway to the front door of the establishment. There was a sign by it that announced toilets, with an arrow pointing off towards the bushes beyond. Unsure whether it was genuine instruction or sarcastic tomfoolery, he opened the door. 'Johnny B. Goode' was playing, and with that, the fifties-diner motif that had been somehow jammed into the unlikely husk of an old hunting lodge was cemented. The inside was more of a shock to the senses – but the biggest shock of all was to find that it somehow worked. The dark wood panelling and stylings, with the ornate architraves, played perfect host – somehow – to the neon signs, beer posters and huge prints of Fatty Arbuckle.

'First time?' came a voice. It was female and close, and Cam turned to a booth that could well have been plucked from a medieval ale house, if it didn't have a huge chandelier of Bud Light bottles overhead. Sat within were two women – the two women he guessed he was here to see. They both looked at him expectantly, as if it was a usual source of mirth, watching people's first reactions to this cultural petri dish.

'Yeah, first time,' Cam said, edging towards the booth. He glanced about, but didn't see another soul. 'I'm Cam Killick,' he said. To his surprise he felt a queasy sense of nerves, as if the people in the booth were famous. To him, he supposed, they were. 'You're the *Norfolk Unexplained* team?'

'The very same,' said the woman on the left. She was dressed in a sharp business suit with a trilby, a black pony-tail swishing beneath the back of the brim. The woman next to her simply nodded. She carried more of the A-level student aesthetic. She wore a T-shirt emblazoned with

Japanese manga characters that Cam had no chance of recognising, under a grey hoodie, a huge pair of earphones slung around her neck. She wore rimless glasses and what he believed younger people called a resting bitch face.

'Gupta and Ferris,' said the woman in the trilby, thumbing first at herself then her apparently furious associate.

Cam slid into the booth. 'Good to meet you. I've … I've listened to all 153 of your episodes.'

'Favourite one?' asked Gupta. Cam could feel Ferris' eyes watching him.

Cam felt put on the spot, and heat rose with a tingle. 'The one with the haunted sheep's head at the Dog Inn, the one that survived the fire with the toy car in its mouth.'

'Good answer,' said Gupta.

'An aficionado,' said Ferris, unblinking. The conversation paused as a waiter arrived. He was wearing a black-and-white refereeing jersey, with hair shining perfect with an oil slick of Brylcreem. He was carrying two of the thickest-looking milkshakes Cam had ever seen. So thick that the straws were standing unaided in the centre of both glasses.

He put them down, while asking Cam, 'Anything for you, sir?'

Before he could answer, Gupta did. 'He'll have the same.' Taken aback, Cam simply nodded. The waiter disappeared, presumably to wedge as much dairy as he possibly could into a similarly sized glass. There was silence while they weighed each other up. It was excruciating, so Cam broke it as quickly as he could. 'Vintage headphones,' he said to Ferris, pointing at the huge headphones. 'You like music?'

Ferris didn't blink. 'Recent studies have shown that foreign crafts only have to breach the earth's exosphere to hijack an ear pod's Bluetooth signal. It used to have to be so much closer – at least the stratosphere, but better still the troposphere. Just to be sure.'

Cam stared dumbly and wished he hadn't opened his mouth.

Ferris continued. 'Easier than ever for aliens to speak directly into our brains.'

Gupta intervened and took the lead again. 'You wanted to ask us about an old case that we covered on the show?'

'That's right,' Cam said. 'The Brindleys.'

'Of course it is.'

'Of course it is,' echoed Ferris. Cam was usually good at reading people, but he was in obscure new territory with them.

'Is that all right?' He found himself asking. He didn't know if he'd already disappointed them, but that was exactly what their reactions suggested.

'We knew as much,' replied Gupta. 'Given the press conference called for later today.'

'How do you mean?' asked Cam.

Gupta took a sip from her straw, but because it was see-through, Cam could see that whatever was in the glass wasn't coming up. However, Gupta played it off as if she'd taken a huge gulp. He genuinely had no idea what to make of these people.

'All journalists have sources, and at heart that's what we are. Journalists. We do the weirdo stuff on the side because we find it interesting, but of course it doesn't pay.'

'Nothing fun ever does,' said Ferris with a world-weariness that suggested she had learned that through experience.

Cam knew the story, knew their background. It was why he came to them. Karishma Gupta and Eleanor Ferris were journalists for the *Eastern Daily Gazette*, the main local newspaper in East Anglia. In that capacity, strange stories would occasionally cross their desks, and eventually they had decided to start the *Norfolk Unexplained* podcast in order to discuss them. It turned out that the region was practically full of mad legends and creepy myths, thanks to its unique landscape and rich history. They seemed to have endless material – and they were utterly hell-bent, they continually proclaimed, on revealing the truth.

'Something's happened, hasn't it?' Gupta asked. 'Some kind of development in the case, surely?'

Cam realised that the information he possessed, and the nature of what he had done, could be very valuable to the podcasters of *Norfolk Unexplained* and their audience – and then doubly useful to them as journalists too.

Was he under any obligation to keep it secret?

No, he decided.

'Yesterday I found the car.'

Gupta's eyes took on the shape and size of ping-pong balls, before she tried to regain her cool – but just as soon as she tried to compose herself, she abandoned all sense of composure altogether.

'You found it?' she asked in a near-euphoric whisper. 'After all this time, some rando comes in and finds the car? No offence.'

Cam had no idea what a rando was and thought it might have something to do with his military background and some play on the character name Rambo. 'None taken.'

'Where was it?'

Cam paused. While he didn't feel any obligation to keep the story completely secret, he didn't want to burn any bridges with Norfolk police and DS Rogers. If the *Norfolk Unexplained* podcast broke the story about the Brindley car, with Cam Killick as the source, Rogers would be furious and keep him out of future developments. This was something he wanted to avoid. 'Can you keep it a secret until after the police make their announcements?'

'Are you joking?' Gupta replied incredulously. 'The mystery car from years ago has been found, and you want us not to report on it.'

Next to her, Ferris was typing frantically on her phone. Cam could imagine her urgently emailing the editorial desk asking them to clear the front page for the story behind the story.

He realised asking these reporters not to report was like asking a bear not to shit in the woods. But he had to try to keep them quiet. If they had resources that could help him get to the bottom of the Brindley matter, he could use all the help he could get. So, he decided to play hardball.

He stood. 'You know, this might not be the best idea after all.'

'Woah, woah, woah,' Gupta said, suddenly panicking. 'You can't just drop a bombshell like that and piss off! You've got to fill in the blanks.'

'What kind of human does that?' added Ferris.

'This one,' Cam said, sticking fast to his guns.

'Stop, stop, stop.' Gupta was standing now too. 'This is one of those situations where we can surely come to some kind of quid pro quo arrangement.'

'With lots of back-and-forth backscratching,' added Ferris.

Cam couldn't quite help himself from grimacing at the thought, but he wanted them to spell it out. 'How exactly could you scratch my back?'

'We have the resources of the rest of the paper, which come in particularly useful, whenever our two passions collide. If one of the stories contains a whiff of the weird, then it works very well for us. That's why we've got all sorts on the Brindley piece for the podcast, because they were covered by the paper – actually covered unironically that is. Unlike some of our other podcast episodes like when some granny announces that the unusually large marrow she's grown who is the work of…'

'Aliens,' finished Ferris.

Cam could understand where she was coming from. The Brindley disappearance was a genuine mystery, packed with real questions that went beyond tall tales and the unexplained.

'We've got contacts, old editions, information, data…'

'Credibility,' added Ferris without a hint of irony.

'And we're more likely to tell the truth than the police. If you want to hear the real story, we can deliver it, warts and all. Not some sanitised version that plays nice on spreadsheets.'

Cam looked at them both. They seemed to know an awful lot, not just about the way the police were handling things – DS Rogers excluded – but about how beneficial it would be for the Brindley matter to get rubber stamped and sailed into the sunset, not least from a PR perspective.

'You've got my attention,' he said. He thought about how every excursion he'd ever been on was based on intel, and how his present well of info had run dry. *Norfolk Unexplained* might be able to fill in an awful lot of background if the right arrangement was struck. 'There's a couple of rules.'

'Oh of course, rules!' Gupta said sarcastically. The shake arrived for Cam, with the same magical upright straw.

'Hold on.' This was where Cam was going to rely on these two podcasters having attributes outside of their jobs as reporters. The very nature of their podcast suggested a love of the odd, a love of the weird, a love of conspiracy – but more than anything else, he thought it suggested a thirst for the truth. 'I can give you the truth. I can give you the inside track, that you will hear only from me.'

He then leaned heavily on the drama and aura that conspiracies carried in popular media. 'I will tell you what nobody else knows. One day, there'll be a time for these things to come out, and you'll be the ones to break it wide open. For the paper or the podcast – you can pick. But it can't be now.' And then the line he thought would be the kicker. '*They* are covering it up. They don't want the public to know.'

He thought this was true, to an extent, but more importantly he thought that if he made out he was some kind of secretive informer, it might make him indispensable to them.

'You'd be our Deep Throat,' Ferris said, burning interest all too evident thanks to her ever-loosening grip on her icy facade.

Cam had always hated that expression but knew it would seal the deal. 'Yours, and yours alone.'

'Prove it.' Gupta said. 'What have you got?'

Cam looked around. All waiters had gone, and they were alone with their stand-off and shakes. He took out his phone and thumbed through to the video he took the day before. He handed it to Gupta. 'Just don't delete it,' he said.

Gupta watched with ever-widening eyes. Even Ferris stood for the first time, leaning across the table top and they held the phone between them.

'I found it yesterday morning at the bottom of Hickling Broad. It was perfect, as you can see. It was verified by the police when they fed the registration number through the DVLA. But nobody was in it. The family was gone.'

'Gone…' whispered Gupta.

Cam had them. 'So, can I trust you both?'

'You can,' said Gupta.

'I knew it was aliens,' said Ferris. She pulled her phone, slid it into the middle of the table, and pressed a large red record button in the centre. 'Continue.'

Cam looked at the phone screen between them, saw a timecode rolling by as it captured the audio in the room. He was about to go on record. No turning back.

Gupta ignored the phone recorder and pressed on. 'What's the latest? Are you inside the investigation?'

Up until twenty-four hours prior, Cam *was* the investigation. And now, with Rogers' encouragement, and the police deciding it was all done and dusted, he guessed it was down to him again. He breathed in and out, and spoke clearly, leaning slightly towards the device on the tabletop. 'I am.'

'Tell us everything,' Gupta said. 'But what do you need from us?'

It didn't take Cam long to tell them exactly what he wanted, after which it took far longer for him to tell the two journalists everything he knew – between sips of a milkshake so heavy a diabetic coma would be a welcome reprieve.

19

The press conference was a queasy monument to an unearned success that wasn't even complete. Rogers' case was paraded for the local media as a triumph for the long-standing dedication of local police officers, after hours – no, years – of tireless work. Rogers had at least been invited to say a few words, as the detective who was in possession of the file at the time of its closure, but she had refused and sat glumly at the back, while the press cameras flashed and their shutters clattered like a pack of excited crows. There was no mention of Cam Killick, which only added to Rogers' sense of injustice.

The glass of wine earlier had done nothing to take the edge off her sorrow. Now that the case was deemed closed, the search for the Brindley family wouldn't continue, and they would now be lost in their Broadland purgatory for evermore.

Chief Inspector Hilton had on his best dress uniform and had even nipped out for a haircut since debriefing Rogers that morning. Rogers thought she could also detect a light layer of stage powder on his forehead, but that might just be wishful thinking. His excitement could barely be contained by the dress uniform, as he stared down the cameras (paying particular attention to the big television lens in the middle of the pack) and told what Rogers knew were flat-out lies. The fact that they were in the station car park under a handful of big tents, since the press room inside hadn't been deemed large enough for such an occasion, didn't detract this from feeling like Norfolk Constabulary's own 'Four Seasons Total Landscaping' moment.

Rylance stood in his own dress uniform off to the side, alongside a couple of media officers and the press liaison.

Preening arseholes, thought Rogers. She was embarrassed once again, but cold fury started to come with it. What ethical police force did this? What officers signed off on this, let alone the chief?

What else was really going on here?

The more she looked at the stage, the more she realised that she could see everyone from the station. It was like the constabulary HQ had been tipped on its head, with everyone who had been inside poured out into the rows in front of her. But that gave her an idea.

She stood and edged out from the row past a couple of people – neither of whom looked at her save to huff at the inconvenience.

She glanced back at the peacocks on the stage. Hilton was in the grip of his adoring public, while Rylance watched her go. She didn't mind that. As long as he didn't follow her.

As soon as she was away from the car park and the canopies of the hasty shelters, she upped the pace. Straight in through the garage door, through the equipment cages, and up the lift. She hit the button for the top floor.

They hadn't even started questions yet, and boy, would Hilton like those. He'd chew over each one with glee. As long as Rylance didn't get suspicious, she was golden.

At least for a short while.

Top floor. Empty. A ghost office. The anterooms for the chief's staff were all dead. Everyone really was downstairs.

She marched down the carpeted aisle to the double doors at the back, seething more with every step.

She no longer cared about her job.

Killick was right. She had taken the money. But if she got fired, at least her conscience would back her up on all those penniless nights to come. Some things, like integrity, weigh more than coins ever could.

She pushed her way into the chief's office and rounded his desk. The aim here was to leave no trace, but she was lucky that she didn't need to search. She'd watched Hilton put the file in the filing cabinet by his desk – top drawer – and when she saw the haircut, she knew straight away that nothing had interfered with preparing for his moment. So the file, the entire Brindley case file that Rogers had kept for so long until that very morning, should still be sitting there.

When she slid open the cabinet drawer, there it was.

Blood tingling, Rogers took it out and wasted no time.

Back out in the top floor office, she found the copier. It was a huge industrial thing that could work magic if used correctly. She knew how to use it, since anything paperwork related was apparently now a core police skill.

It just depended how much time it took.

She opened the folder to start, but noticed something was different about it. It took a moment for her to work out what it was, and she turned it in her hands to look at it from different angles.

Then it hit her.

It was heavier.

Noticeably.

She checked the clock, then quickly leafed through the stack.

She was so stunned, she almost couldn't think. One word pierced through the mental short-circuit.

Bastards.

She was intimately aware of every detail of the file, every page and hand-scrawled note, but now as she flicked through, she found things in this four-decade old file that she'd never seen before. Now the case was closed, more detail had been added.

Added … or returned?

There were charts she didn't recognise, statements she hadn't seen, new photographs.

Her blood boiled.

The imaginary stink of injustice hit her nostrils again.

She was resolute now. She would continue searching for the Brindley family. And Tommy Brindley. That melancholy boy she knew would never leave his sister's side. She would conduct her own investigation, career be damned.

She put the first sheet in and checked the clock over the exit. She was sure she had time, but looking at the new weight of the file, it would be close.

She hit the green button and held her breath.

20

Cam parked on the edge of Hickling, on the sparse gravel of a boatyard's empty car park. Judging by its silence and the blank stare of the windows, the workers had long since been dismissed and a lone motion-activated security light was now his only guide.

'Now, you're gonna have to sleep here for a bit,' he said, turning to Nala as soon as the engine was off. He glanced around the dark corners next to the huge riverside ware-house, itself in a state of merry disrepair. He didn't know what Nala understood of them pulling up in a darkened car park like this, but he assumed she had an inkling that he was going underwater soon. She had been bankside at every one of his dives since he adopted her, name and all, as a puppy. He ruffled the fur at the back of her ears. Going off on an ill-advised solo dive in the middle of the night, without even his dog for company, didn't sit too well with him.

Cam ushered Nala between the seats and into the back of the van, Velcro-ed his dryrobe tight and got out. Opening the sliding door, he saw Nala hunkering down obediently in a dog bed between the shelves, tanks, fins and regulators, while he unzipped the duffel bag he'd packed earlier, and checked its contents.

Everything was just as he had left it. A single tank, regulator, fins, mask, his Sola dive torch, it all looked back up at him from between the teeth of the parted zip. Satisfied, he zipped it back up, threw the whole thing on his back and slid the door shut. He locked the car with a keyless clunk and marched out of the boatyard, into the darkness and up to the main road.

If this was going to work, secrecy and anonymity were crucial. The thugs' words from last night echoed in his ears, and their blows rang in his head.

It took ten minutes to walk the half-mile back up to the track. It was now cordoned off with a single strip of police tape. In terms of a deterrent, it was weak at best and looked more like a finish line than something that would keep someone out. He hadn't seen a single car on the walk and, as he ducked under the tape and marched down the blackness of the muddy track into the trees, Cam felt confident that he'd got away with it.

After another half an hour, he got to the site, and took a moment to stand and admire it. He'd be forgiven for thinking that nothing had happened there at all. Any hint of commotion was gone, all suggestion of yesterday's drama long since blown away or swallowed by the intervening drizzle. Through the gap in the foliage, the water stared at him, a vast, near-flawless mirror of obsidian. It promised him solace, but also a cold edge of mystery. His body and mind longed for it, yearning for the reassuring grasp that only the underwater world could give.

Cam stood on the bank, listening to the softest breeze rush through the trees. Reeds wobbled gently, as if brushed by a ghostly deity.

Rogers had said it herself – the case was over. All searches called off. There couldn't possibly have been enough time for the police and their dive teams to properly scour the broad for clues in the time before they were sent home.

And Cam had been down there. He'd seen the lay of the land, knew the underwater terrain. Properly and effectively conducting a full underwater search was a slow, laborious and painstaking process – he'd been on enough underwater search and recovery missions to know that the police hadn't put nearly enough time into searching this site. The previous day had left him hell-bent on finding answers, and if those answers weren't coming anytime soon up on land, they might well be found down there, where past and present collided. Added to the fact that there was now the dank whiff of corruption in the air, he felt he had no choice.

More than any of this, Cam was convinced. Emboldened. None of this was an accident, he was sure of that now. This was murder and conspiracy, and it was time to go back into the water, to look for something – *anything* – they had missed. Cam knew the water couldn't lie. Those kids flashed in his head, that famous final picture of them, tired, being ushered down those stone steps at the mayor's house. So many people had failed them – but Cam wouldn't.

He dropped his dryrobe from his shoulders, his wetsuit already on. His boots were swapped for flippers, the tank tossed on his back and fastened tight, and he strapped the multipurpose dive torch to the back of his hand, a genius product quirk that allowed him to be hands-free while underwater. His mask was given a quick rinse with a mixture of saliva and a splash from the broad itself, before he yanked it on and walked into the black heart of the huge body of water. His extremities immediately chilled, but the shock was soon replaced by the buzz of a need about to be sated. Within seconds, he was up to his chest, his shoulders, his chin, and then, at last, his head disappeared under the surface.

The relief of the water's close embrace swept in, and he felt all anxiety, all the stinging needles of pressure pull back and fade. His breathing began to settle and he found the perfect rhythm. The dark pressed tight into his mask, but it didn't give him fear. The water was his domain, his sanctuary.

Cam switched on the torch on the back of his hand and rotated the settings around to floodlight mode. A fat cone of light burned into the brown murk in front of him. Silver fish, caught on the edge of the illumination, retreated into darker territories and weeds danced like the skeletal spectres of trees long drowned. He knew exactly where he was going and followed near enough the same course he had taken yesterday. That said, even if this was all new, the way would have been rendered obvious by the pressed silt and disturbed rocks that betrayed a dull trail across the bottom.

There was no life to speak of now except for a lone pike. Half a metre long, it split across his vision like a green dart, its two black eyes never leaving him, like a painting in a pub whose stare would remain forever unbroken no matter where you sat.

He had about an hour in his tank, which should be enough for a thirty-metre search radius if the bottom remained clear and visibility remained at a similar level — which was about two metres ahead.

His plan was simple. Head down, eyes on the bottom, hand over hand, easing himself along. He hadn't bothered with his flippers so that he wouldn't go too fast, and he allowed his neoprene-covered toes to nudge the silt softly.

Within a few moments, he found them — those four aged depressions where the car's tyres had rested for thirty years.

The place looked bereft and ghostly — the only suggestion that something huge had happened there being the marks in the silt and the memories held by the water itself. The four tyre treads sat fifteen centimetres deep, and there around them, were footprints of a much fresher kind, some even bearing the sole detail of the dive team the day before. Cam moved into the middle of the four indentations and hovered in the exact position the car had come to rest all those years ago.

The eeriness came to him in waves, but it never dented his control. He felt cool and calm despite the peculiarity of the setting, and he waved the torch at the area around his feet. The only thing he noticed that garnered any kind of interest was the scratched-out crawl marks of crustaceans who had moved on now their shelter had gone. Aside from this observation, however, nothing seemed out of place.

Starting on this central spot, he kept the torch on the floor and began a slow spin, staring intently at the bottom of the broad with every rotation. He went wider in radius until he had to move with the beam, and soon he was swimming in widening circles, his gaze and torch beam never leaving the dirt. It was a tactic taught in the old diver reconnaissance training, for when he was dispatched to pull things from the mud. He'd been given full understanding of how an underwater crime scene worked — and he had worked a lot of them since. One option was a grid search, but that was best when you had a lot of time, and an equally large amount of manpower. When you were alone, an ever-widening spiral search was always preferable, since it offered a lone pair of eyes a thoroughness through simple geometric coverage. Cam never thought about being part of a team anymore, so swimming in circles was always what he ended up doing.

After five minutes of careful, methodical trawl, he checked his readings. Air consumption was spot-on. By keeping it slow and calm, he was in control of his exertions, and therefore didn't expend a high amount of oxygen. He should get another forty-five minutes from here, possibly up to an hour.

He pressed on.

He was about ten metres from the car's original resting site when he encountered something strange – a smallish patch of knotweed that somehow hadn't died in the chill. Using his right hand to angle the torch at the clump, he bent down and ran his hand through it.

He damn near pissed his wetsuit, when an eye looked back at him between the drifting fronds. His heart wanted to jump clear through the neoprene.

Oh god, I've found one of them.

But sense quickly prevailed, as he composed himself. Black and shiny, with an off-white surround, it looked false, cartoonish and out of place. He cleared the debris with a finger, and as the tendrils of weed unravelled, a second eye appeared next to it. Then a tiny face emerged, and a snout. Gently, he pulled out a child's teddy, a little dog with big floppy ears and huge tired eyes. An embroidered tongue poked out from beneath its nose.

Cam's stomach dropped as he fought off the urge to jump to conclusions.

He brushed away some of the silt to reveal brown fur and held the thing at arm's length, scrutinising it once more, a connection to history making his hand sing.

He couldn't help it now; his mind crackled with the question. *Why had it not been found yesterday?* Did the dive teams miss it, or – he thought as the echo of Rogers' new orders rang in his ears – had they been ordered to get the car out, then leave anything else they'd found where it was?

He put the dog in a pouch on his waist, raised the torch and continued to search – all the while thoughts racing through his head with unchecked abandon. This was a protected area. Next to zero boat traffic. And while he would like to believe this toy could have been dropped by any child, he just couldn't ignore his instinct. This dog could well be evidence that Hannah Brindley, the youngest child, had been here. In the water.

Cam continued to search for another half an hour, while painful images of Hannah's last moments jack-in-the-boxed in his head – then, suddenly, something bright flirted at the corner of his vision. It was coming from above his head. He glanced up, expecting to see a fish, its underbelly having been caught in his torch glare. There was only darkness above.

He waited a second, and there it was again. A light, moving, side to side.

Oh *no*.

Cam reached for his own torch and switched it off, punching himself into darkness except for that one source of light, casting about, flitting overhead.

He couldn't move. He held his breath, even though he knew he shouldn't.

Overhead, dancing across the surface, unmistakable now, was another searching torchlight.

21

Cam's hands hung limply at his sides, anxiety fizzing the blood in his veins. Overhead, the torch spotlight swept across the vast surface, chasing only a metre above his crown.

His paranoia urgently filled in blanks. Someone was on the bank, looking for him. Someone knew he was there.

He tilted his quivering wrist to look at his watch face and checked his readings. He had enough air for fifteen minutes, at an absolute push. He needed a plan.

Wait it out and hope the person above decides they've got it wrong and moves on? But if they found his bag, he'd still have to explain himself. The two parties would still meet. Cam, in the long run, wouldn't get away with anything.

Another option would be to swim into the middle of the water and pop up when his air ran out. He turned and looked into the deep belly of the broad. Without the glow of his torchlight, he couldn't see a thing. The consistency of the water was too stout to offer anything but the promise of dark nothingness for acres. He knew, if he started swimming that way, it would feel like forever. And he knew from experience that when you were down to your last few moments of air, those moments sprinted quicker than wildfire.

It had been drilled into Cam, through endless training and experience, to always give himself the strongest chance of survival – and the chance to fight another day. As he peered into the black, he thought staying put was his best bet. He would wait it out for as long as he possibly could. He started to run a rhythmic breathing incantation in his head.

Breathe in for three.

Hold for five.

Out for eight.

Cam leaned into the rhythm and tried to get as low as he could, almost sitting now. Staying still would bring the cold in quicker than a burglar on a footballer's away trip, so he kept his hands just about warm through soft, circular motions of his wrists. The same with his ankles for his feet. Every six repetitions of his breathing mantra, he rotated his shoulder blades. Three times forward, three times back.

His focus became resolute, all-encompassing. This was a test of nerve, resolve and steel, as he fought against his body's requirements and the ticking clock of an air tank with a dwindling supply.

Cam could see nothing except the sweep of the torch and the pictures his mind painted of men on the bank, convinced he was there, but unable to locate him.

It all conspired to fire something in Cam – something he didn't know he had anymore. It was the same feeling from last night, though he was more in control today. A burning will to see justice. For the Brindleys. For the little girl whose stuffed dog he'd plucked from the mulch of this ungodly resting place.

Cam was going to give this a damn good go.

In for three.

Hold for five.

Out for eight.

Make your body believe that's all it needs. Dare your body to use less.

And in that moment, he took a cold thrill from another realisation – that he'd been taking the lead and tackling the odds, without the aid of his meds. He was underwater, granted, which was the only place he ever felt truly at peace anymore. But these were abnormal circumstances with unexpected pressures – and he was *thriving*.

In a way.

He hadn't fallen to pieces, put it that way.

Not yet.

The seconds rolled and minutes passed. The torch was omnipresent it seemed, its beam skating the surface with almost the same consistency as Cam's breathing pattern – until, at last, it stopped moving. He watched the disc over his head, frozen in place with a predatory stillness. Then abruptly, it disappeared. The black rushed in, but Cam refused to move.

He checked his regulator. He had about 3 per cent of his air left in the tank. He'd managed to stretch those initial fifteen minutes out to twenty-two. It had, in a strange way, flown by – but he wouldn't get out yet. He wanted to give himself the best chance of being alone when he emerged and couldn't be sure the danger had cleared.

Counting down the seconds slavishly, he sought to elongate the gap between each one. The lengths of the seconds doubled, until he was down to 2 per cent, then 1 per cent. The torch beam didn't reappear, and his time was up. He had no choice.

With his own torch beam still off, Cam ascended to the surface and gently broke through. He felt freezing air on the top of his head as his mask broke through next, and he could see. His eyes were fully adjusted to the darkness already and, thanks to the moonlight, he could make out shapes and outlines on the bank. From his position, twenty metres out, it looked clear. He spat out the mouthpiece and breathed fresh air which seared his lungs, stiff as a shot of bleach. Keeping as much of himself below the water-line as he could, Cam did a gentle breaststroke towards the bank, his eyes scanning his exit. With every stroke forward, more detail was added to the sight ahead – and still he couldn't see anybody. He emerged slowly out of the water, trying not to splash, and edged up to the mud of the bankside opening.

He paused, his senses crackling. He scrutinised the trees so hard his eyes began to ache.

Please, he thought, *please let my bag be there.* Walking back down the track in all this soaking kit on this late November evening was a prospect unappetising at best.

He would do it though. He knew he would. He was in survival mode now.

Cam carried on, heading out of the broad towards where his bag was hidden against the roots of a gnarled tree stump, when his instinct was snagged by the conviction that something wasn't right.

In an instant, with the water lapping against his shins, Cam froze. He tried again to stare into the body of the trees but only saw the outlines of the bushes softly moving this way and that. He peered intently.

Wait, Cam's senses screamed.

One of the shapes wasn't moving. While the rest slowly rolled with the breeze, one stayed stiff, straight and steady.

Just as his eyes started to focus in on the stationary figure, the centre of the dark shape exploded in a ball of light. Cam was blinded by a sudden, focused torch beam and the silent night was cut in half by a deep male voice.

'You must be fucking freezing.'

October 1987

This one is worse than ever. I've never heard shouting like it. Dad sounds like something is going to break loose from inside him, like a piece of his voice might snap off and drift away. Mum is pleading with him to calm down, and all he seems to do is find different ways of telling her she doesn't understand.

'Maud, you don't get it. It's gone!' Dad screams now from inside the office. 'All of it.'

I'm sitting on the stairs at Brindley Hall. I know I should call it home by now, but it just doesn't feel like it. It's not like our old house in Thetford, with the bright little kitchen and the bedroom that me and Tommy shared. *That* was a home.

I look through the banister supports, my fingers tracing the little faces in the whirls of the wood's surface. I've found one that looks like a golden retriever. I'm going to look at it every day. My brother sits two steps above me, and every time the noise goes from horrible to scary, he puts a hand on my shoulder.

He is my hero.

'But you don't do that!' shouts Mum. 'Or at least, you told me you didn't?'

I imagine Mum standing over Dad in his office chair as it faces that computer of his. He keeps calling it 'the apple', but it doesn't look anything like a bit of fruit.

'I don't!' Dad shouts back. 'But I've told a lot of other people to. A lot. Some of them are very important. This is bad, Maud.'

On the word bad, Tommy rubs my shoulder again. I turn to look at him, and he rolls his eyes and purses his lips, just like Mum does when she's fed up with something that keeps happening but she's trying to make it funny. I know what Tommy is doing. He's trying to make me feel better.

'Well, didn't you know this could happen?' Mum says, and I tense. I can feel Tommy has held his breath too.

You must never make it Dad's fault, Mum.

Dad doesn't like that.

I hear a clatter, as if a chair has fallen over, then stomping feet, and all I can imagine is Dad marching at Mum with that mad look he often gets – but suddenly I feel a hand on my shoulder.

'Enough of this nonsense, let's go and play somewhere else.'

Tommy takes my hand, and I let him guide me away.

22

Cam remained silent but reached up to get his mask out of the way, before looping it securely round his arm. He shrugged off the tank, let it drop into the mud with a wet thud. The fight or flight flame had been ignited in him once more, and again it was the former that burned brighter. 'If you've come here for a spot of dogging, you've got your night-time woods mixed up. Identify yourself.'

'I'm not sure I'll be doing that,' chuckled the voice, still from behind the glare of the torch. It was a voice he was unfamiliar with, but he still wracked his brain for a match. Cam wasn't sure just how much threat the man posed, but wasn't going to take it lightly. He maintained a steady course as he exited the water. 'I don't know how you guys do it,' the voice continued. 'Bloody mad, the lot of you.'

Cam detected age in the voice. An inflection; gravel and confidence in every word.

'You should give it a try sometime,' said Cam as he emerged fully on to the bank. 'Mind if I get dry? And if that light starts to shake, and it turns out you're beating one off, I'm telling everybody.'

Whether it was thanks to the burning hurt he felt for Hannah Brindley or his growing sense of self-control, he didn't know, but Cam felt somehow *empowered*. It wasn't all that different from when he was on excursions with the SBS, like he was firing up old machinery again, watching it juddering tentatively back to life. He felt, for the first time in as long as he could remember, a bit like the old Cam. The Cam that could make a damn good go of any situation, and back himself to come out on top every time.

'Yes, I think you better get warmed up,' said the voice. 'Can't have you perishing on me before we've got to the good stuff.'

'Are you armed?' Cam asked.

'I could put a hole in your heart any second and you wouldn't know where it came from.'

'And you're not talking bollocks?'

The darkness was cracked by the brittle click of a gun's hammer being cocked.

Despite the jump in Cam's heartbeat, he forced himself not to pause as he moved towards the familiar tree stump, as unflustered as he could. 'Is my bag where I left it?'

'I'm not interested in your bag.'

At least that's something. Cam walked to the rotten stump, behind which, sure enough, was his bag. He took out the towel, unwrapped his mask from his arm and tossed it in. He unzipped the back seam of his wetsuit with an oft-practised gesture, the glare lighting up his skin with such clarity he could see the goosebumps rise, and steam pump out into the night air. 'Do you mind?' he said with overt irritation.

'Oh, forgive me,' said the voice, thick with sarcasm. Nevertheless, the torch clicked off. 'Don't try anything. You wouldn't make it far in any case.'

Cam took the whole suit off and dried himself in the darkness. 'Do you mind telling me what this is about?' he asked. 'Or are you just putting the exclamation mark on your thugs' message from last night?'

'Ah they've already found you, have they? That would make sense I suppose.'

Two interested parties, thought Cam. *This just gets better and better. And who the hell is 'they'?*

'Your recent swimming trips really have opened up Pandora's box.'

Cam pulled his T-shirt over his head, the dry cotton immediately a relief from the damp chill. 'So, you're someone else who'd rather I'd never found the car and the whole thing went away, right?'

The man didn't answer for a long while, but when he did, his tone had adopted a more acidic edge. 'Your attitude doesn't suggest you're taking this very seriously. I'm telling you now, you should.'

The near-banter they'd been exchanging just moments before had gone. These words carried deep bite. Cam laughed with defiance, but he knew it was hollow. 'Or you'll kill me, right? Something dramatic like that?'

'There are other things that are equally as persuasive. Sometimes more.'

Cam dragged the dryrobe around his shoulders. 'So, what happens if I don't listen, and I keep cracking on, and I find something you don't like?'

'This gun here, this primitive tool is just to keep you in place. I don't need violence to ruin a man's life. Some things are bigger than sticks and stones.'

This settled any lingering doubts Cam had. Last night's visitors had relied on brute thuggery. This man's approach was different. Measured. Controlled. The voice carried a snake-like charm and manipulation, one that Cam associated with those from the upper echelons of society.

Cam was sure now. There were two different parties in play.

He leant into his assumption about the kind of man he was dealing with tonight. 'So, why do you have any interest in this? The Brindley case is tabloid fodder, isn't it? Small change for someone of your obvious *power* – which, to me, sounds like a bucket of bullshit.'

Cam could hear the snarl on the man's face as he replied. 'I know you live alone with a little dog called Nala, a Shih Tzu-cross, and which vet you take the mutt to for shots. I know your inside leg measurement in fatigues, wetsuit and dress uniform. I know exactly what you've been doing in places like Mozambique and Rhode Island, and just how riddled you are with PTSD. It's rotting you from the inside out. I know how many confirmed kills are on your record, and how many are not. I know what tablets you're taking, where you get them from, and how many times you wake up in the night wishing you'd have a heart attack to put you out of your misery. I know about the breakdown off the coast of Somalia, and I know what to do to make it happen again.'

Cam was too stunned to reply, his mouth suddenly bone dry.

'I know where your parents are, where your sister is, where your grandparents are buried. Cameron Killick, believe me, I know everything about you. *Everything.*'

'Prove it.'

'Your parents are in the Cotswolds, your sister's in Montreal, and your grandparents are buried together in a place called Hathersage – which sounds very lovely I might add.'

'So you've got some paperwork, who gives a shit?'

'Rhode Island was off-the-books. But I still know you arrived via rigid inflatable boat from Montauk, across

134

Block Island Sound. Traditional SBS team of four, there and back. No loss of life for you boys, but I know the operation was a balls-up and you had to *deposit* a couple of ne'er do wells in Buzzards Bay.'

Cam was stunned. As far as he was aware only six people knew that story, four of those being himself and his unit. This meant serious power, of the highest station. This revealed they had access to his military file, his doctor's surgery records, his outpatient mental health history, even access to databases like animal vaccinations. He'd only told doctors and therapists these most sensitive, private details, which the man trotted out like they were banal entries on a spreadsheet.

Cam was no dummy. In the forces, they had a saying about questionable orders: if they sounded political, they most likely *were* political.

'What does the government want with me?' Cam asked, although he could feel his bravado faltering. He'd been lain so bare it burned. He hated what he'd just heard. Even though he'd made uneasy peace with who he now was, when put so directly, he still couldn't believe that person was him.

'You need to get dry, get home and find a new hobby,' the voice said. 'Forget the car. Stop digging. Step away. Or things will start going very badly for you indeed.'

'I think I've heard enough,' said another voice from somewhere to Cam's right. Cam turned to look, casting about in the dark. He couldn't see anything, and although he wasn't overly familiar with it, he felt he recognised this new voice. Local, for a start, packed with those rolling vowels – and sure enough, out of the track and into the clearing stepped a man Cam knew. Something long glistened in the moonlight, a tube from the man's midriff. A shotgun, raised and ready. Over his head floated a halo of grey made platinum by the blue glow from the sky.

Johnjo Tabernacle.

'You're both trespassing,' he said. 'This is private land and I'll defend it with force if I have to.'

The man in the trees barked back. 'This is just a chat, nothing more.'

'I don't care if you're inviting him round to play tiddly-winks with your missus, you don't do it here.'

'I'm armed. You're in over your head, old fella. This is far bigger than you – or him. If you have any sense, you'll march back down that track now, taking the shells out of that old blunderbuss, and you too will go ahead and forget everything about Hickling Broad and the water here.'

'Ah, you see, you've said it now,' said Tabernacle. Cam still couldn't see his face, just the bobbing of that mane of hair as he spoke. 'Anything to do with Hickling Broad is my business. You see, I'm the custodian of these parts. If you want to see the *formal documentation* asserting that fact, we can do that over a beer somewhere. If you want to quibble some more, pissing about in them willows, be my guest – but it's likely to be a short conversation.'

'You're shooting nobody, old man.'

'Is that so? Sure of that, are you?' Tabernacle waggled the shotgun ominously and pointed it in the direction of the voice.

Cam was impressed. Neither of them knew for sure whether the man was armed but Tabernacle was happy to call his bluff. Even though he couldn't see any of the older man's features, Cam nodded his gratitude.

'Big mistakes are being made here,' said the man in the trees. 'Mistakes you're going to regret.'

'Oh, whoop de do,' said Tabernacle. 'Come on out the trees and be on your way. I'll keep the light off so we don't see you, bogeyman.'

After a moment, the stand-off was broken by twigs snapping and a shape emerging from the trees. The snapping rustle of undergrowth turned to squelching footsteps on muddy grass as the man came across the clearing to the track, right between Tabernacle and Cam.

'Bumpkin, fucking idiots,' he said, walking into the moonlight. Cam caught sight of a square head with hair swept to one side. He had a stocky frame, with a heavy gait and an upright stiffness, adding to Cam's perception that the man was quite a bit older than he was.

Tabernacle turned to watch him go. 'Your car is still by the road,' he said. 'If you fancy doing anything else in secret, try not to be so obvious about it next time.'

'You won't see anything coming next time,' the man replied, almost to himself, but the breeze brought it straight to Cam's ears, a phantom of threat on the wind.

Abruptly, Tabernacle switched the torch on and pointed it at the floor between his and Cam's feet. Now lit by the soft glare of the torchlight, Tabernacle was exactly as Cam remembered him, right down to the same shirt and tie – like he had it in a glass case by his bed ready to break in and don in case of emergency. 'Thank you,' Cam said.

'You're a daft bugger, aren't you,' said Tabernacle. 'Come on, let's get you dry.'

Cam found himself smiling. He drew up the towel around his shoulders and followed – but not before putting the dive pouch containing the stuffed dog into his holdall and zipping it up tight.

23

Tabernacle's home was everything Cam expected, and at the same time a total surprise. It was in the middle of nowhere, down a track off one of the minor roads that ran through the farmland surrounding Hickling. It was little more than a muddy tunnel of hedges, with no signs nor indication there was even a dwelling down there. It was small, secluded, the very definition of hidden away, and when they arrived in the pitch black it was like stepping into a previous century. Cam caught the burly shape of a thatched roof overhead as he followed Tabernacle up the scuffed front path.

Inside, after a couple of moments of Tabernacle clomping about with a long taper, every corner of the building became washed in the orange flicker-glow of candlelight. Cam could slowly see that antiques hung from the ceiling, sat on the walls, loomed in corners and ruminated on tables all over a carpet so threadbare it was the soft furnishing equivalent of a comb over.

The main theme was an obvious devotion to early cinema. Tabernacle was an avid collector of all things silver screen. Even next to where Cam sat, on a sofa that looked like a Hollywood golden age film agent's casting couch with its faded red velvet upholstery, stood a miniature cine film projector, its lines filmed by dust, betraying its present usage as nothing more than an ornament.

'You've lived here a long time?' Cam asked, taking it all in.

'All my life,' replied Tabernacle, at last slowing down and heading towards a nearby chair. 'Not many houses like these left, I can tell you. You can be here, and nobody would even know you existed.'

Nala sat on Cam's knee and hadn't left him since he got back to the van, panting with excitement at the prospect of more people, and more fuss. Opposite him, under a framed poster for *The Valley of Gwangi*, sat Johnjo Tabernacle himself. His face was flushed, which could have been down to the chill – or down to the fact that in his left hand was a bottle of blended malt.

On his knee sat the shotgun. The men faced each other and sat wordless for a couple of moments. It was the older man that broke the silence.

'Are you going to let this go?' He asked. 'Or am I going to have to put a padlock gate over the old track entrance?'

Cam opted to play negotiator. 'Look,' he said. 'I'm sorry. I don't mean to trespass or take the … take advantage, but things have gone to pieces since I found that car. The police are formally disavowing the whole thing, saying it's case closed. They've told the media the same thing. Everyone now thinks the mystery is solved, and we can pat each other on the back for a job well done.' Cam sat back. He felt hot and bold. 'You were with me yesterday. You saw that there were no bodies. As a custodian, you can't be happy about that. There are so many questions that could be directed at the people you represent. Surely you want to get to the bottom of this just as much as I do.'

The old man looked stone-faced, and merely poured more spirit into his mug. 'I saw the news. They're saying it's case closed and a job well done.'

But Cam was on the kind of old-school roll that used to be so second nature to him. 'Look, Johnjo. There are people who don't want this to come out. Two separate parties. The police too, they want it swept away under the carpet. But why? What are they so scared of?'

Cam was thinking specifically of the teddy he had plucked from the bottom of Hickling Broad. The children that had surely been in the water, then never seen again. Tabernacle began to look unhappy, as if he too would rather everything went away. He topped up his mug for the umpteenth time and spoke again.

'The Brindleys were a family everybody knew, but you never bumped into them quietly. You'd see them out and about, but everything was a performance.'

At the word *performance*, Cam looked up at the movie poster behind Tabernacle. At the bottom was a woman in a showgirl-cowboy crossover outfit, waving to a huge crowd from the back of a horse.

That's what all this felt like now, Cam thought with unhappy irony. The whole Brindley affair was a circus.

He let his eyes come down and rest on Tabernacle. 'You knew them?' he asked.

'Hardly,' Tabernacle snorted. 'But they sure made themselves known. You couldn't pick up a newspaper without a story about them up to some twaddle or other.'

Cam paused for a moment, before thinking *sod it*. 'And then there's you Johnjo, with your remit to protect that water at all costs.' He glanced at the gun in Tabernacle's lap with a nod. 'You'd be forgiven for thinking that you want that secret hidden too.'

This seemed an affront too far for Tabernacle. He looked like he was about to explode when Cam put both hands up out in front of him in peace. 'Or at least your employer,' he squeezed in. Tabernacle settled back into his chair.

'I'm not questioning your motivations Johnjo – I think there's something going on here that we are both in the dark about. We need to share intel. Two heads are better than one and all that. You know all about me – I'm just some poor idiot who was looking for a purpose and found the wrong one. So come on, how did you get to be the custodian of Hickling Broad on that precise side of the water?'

Tabernacle looked as if he was about to slip into another stubborn mute spell, so Cam ripped the Velcro tab on the dive pouch he'd brought in with him for safekeeping. Any tank could be replaced from his van, any bit of kit could be bought again. What could never be re-salvaged was the artefact from the silt at the bottom of Hickling.

He pulled out the teddy and let it sit in the palm of his hand. 'I found this out there tonight. Where the Brindley car was found. Do you see how wrong this picture is?'

Tabernacle stared at the item in wonder. He looked how Cam had felt when he found the car. A piece of history supposedly lost, pulled from the fabric of time, into the present.

'Something more is going on,' said Cam. 'If the teddy was in the water, the girl most likely was too. This isn't some runaway family, hiding an old car to cover their tracks. There were supposed to be two kids in that car and after finding this, I can't rest until I find out where they are and what happened to them.'

Tabernacle's brow unmeshed, and his countenance opened with it. Yes, protecting your employer's interests was always a noble thing – but some matters were of a far greater importance.

Tabernacle coughed to clear his throat, and fixed his gaze on the shotgun as, finally, he spoke. 'I was known locally at the time, you could say. I suppose they saw me as someone in the area that people would listen to. I'd done a bit of local glad-handing with the parish council, bits and pieces and all that, and they knew from my stint as a gamekeeper that I'm handy with telling people to bugger off. So I was offered a lifetime deal with a cash payout every year.'

Cam felt excitement with even this slight progress. 'Paid out by the estate? The Belvedere Estate?' asked Cam.

'That's right. They explained that they owned bits of the water and the land on that side of the broad. They wanted someone to keep an eye on the place because they weren't from around here. It was an investment that they wanted some security for. That was my understanding.'

'But did they ever tell you why that land was so important?'

'Never,' said Tabernacle, and Cam thought he began to look a little bashful. 'I feel stupid for not asking now, but it never came up. It was just a good gig at the time. For me it was a bit of a retirement package. Of course, when I agreed to it all them years ago, that fee I got paid used to go a long way. Now, with the cost of living the way it is, it buys a few beers during the quieter months, but that's about it. Besides, I barely had to do anything before this week – then you came along.'

'I need to ask this honestly and forgive me for doing so,' Cam said. 'But did you know or suspect that car was down there?'

Tabernacle looked at him with pleading resignation. 'No, I did not.'

'OK. Did you ever meet the Brindleys in any way?'

'Not directly, although they didn't live a million miles from here. They bought that Feather House, which was a beautiful old home out near Thrigby.'

Cam frowned. 'Feather House? I thought they lived at Brindley Hall?'

'That's what they renamed it to, when Freddie Brindley decided to give his ego a stretch. It never took on with the locals.'

Cam thought about that, an idea forming. He held it to one side for the moment. 'So, is there anything at all you can tell me about them?'

The older man looked at Cam with a protruding bottom lip for a long moment. Abruptly, he put down his mug and stood. 'Hang on,' he said, before leaving the room and Cam in that chintzy mausoleum to long-past movie magic.

A couple of minutes passed as Cam let his eyes wander over the assembled memorabilia when Tabernacle returned and dropped a handful of newspapers in Cam's lap.

'Yes,' Tabernacle said, as he retook his seat with a sigh. Cam took the top paper and unfolded it. The front-page splash of the *Eastern Daily Gazette* read *Socialite Family Disappears*, and beneath was a picture of all four of them. It was one Cam immediately recognised from the newspaper clippings he'd seen from when the Brindleys were finally declared missing. A family snap, four smiles, standing on the deck of a pleasure cruiser. The sun was shining, teeth were gleaming; they were the poster-family for familial perfection.

'Everyone knew them,' Tabernacle continued, with an obvious distaste. 'Or should I say knew *of* them. They moved out here. It's cheaper to buy big flashy homes in Norfolk than it is in more popular postcodes. Or at least, it was. So, they weren't of local stock or anything. It was strange having people come into the area and be so bloody *bold* about it. They were a mad old breed, a lot like the people you see about today. They loved the cameras, loved being in the limelight, in the papers and such. Everything seemed a blessed photo opportunity. Always wanted everything to be about them but forgot what was important.'

'What makes you say that?' asked Cam.

'Ah, well, nothing in particular. Just that they had those kids at home, but the parents were always out on the razzle-dazzle. Young kids too. They didn't know how lucky they were.'

Considering these people had been dead for almost forty years, Cam found it a rather pointed observation. His eyebrows rose in question, one that Tabernacle answered without further prompt.

'They just couldn't have been very good parents, that's all.'

Cam folded the top paper back up and began to open the second one. 'You kept these, all this time?' he asked.

'Bit of a newspaper collector,' Tabernacle replied. 'Only the *Gazette*. I've got everything back there from the moon landings, to 9/11, to King Charles' coronation.'

As Cam opened the second newspaper, he felt a pressure change in the pit of his guts. This headline read: *Brindleys' Last Photo*, with the subheading, *Where did they go after leaving the mayor's house?*

This was the famous one, the image that had forever been entwined with the mystery, both inseparable and indelible – but Cam had never seen it in such detail, and took it in for what felt like the first time. This wasn't one of the low-resolution images that had been uploaded years ago to the internet. No, this was a blown-up print copy, the colours and details all unfaded by the technological limitations of the early internet years. The picture was dark, a night-time shot, of the four walking down some steps. They seemed to be moving at speed, going off the slight hint of motion blur, and headed towards that fated green Jaguar visible at the bottom of the photo. It was a fascinating, haunting insight into those final moments.

Freddie looked harassed, eyes dead, jaw set. Like leaving was a priority. Maud was just behind him, head bowed, focused on every step. She was holding Hannah's hand – who was looking at the camera. The picture of innocence was heart-rending. Cam felt she was looking straight at him. *Solve this*, she seemed to plead with him from the aged print. '*Find me.*'

Cam's heart felt like it was pumping hot and heavy, almost nauseously. That poor girl. Moments away from … what?

Then behind them, keeping his dark blazer tight together as he walked, was the boy, Tommy. It had to be Tommy, but Cam couldn't see his face because he was looking back up the steps. Cam followed his eyeline, back up to the house – and in the corner of the frame spotted a man half in shadow, wearing a dark suit. Was he part of what was to come?

He thought of the two front-page pictures, and how different they were.

The bright, beaming holiday snap, then the bleakly unforgiving image of a family on the cusp of tragedy.

He had to close the top newspaper, because Hannah's eyes boring into him were getting too much for him. 'So what do we do now?'

'I honestly don't know,' replied Tabernacle. 'You've created such a puckaterry around this. This is a quiet corner of the world, Cam. Nobody looks at us twice. I didn't quite realise how much I enjoyed that until this week. For the good of everybody — myself included — I reckon you should think about letting this go.'

Cam had no idea what a puckaterry was, and wondered if it was something you could eat. Still, he looked at the older man as if he'd gone bananas. 'I can't. We still don't have any answers. In that car was a family — a wife, a husband and two kids. If what happened to them was not an accident, then the people responsible have gotten away with it all this time… I can't live with that. Could *you* live with that?'

Tabernacle looked like he had an itch at the base of his spine that was suddenly immensely uncomfortable. He shifted in his seat. 'Don't switch this round on me, I'm just a little old man given a job to do.'

'Don't give me that,' Cam chuckled. 'You may be seventy-odd but you're six foot four and built like a steel outbuilding. I pictured you'd be housed in a garage alongside tractors, not this quaint little cottage.'

They sat in silence for a couple of moments, allowing the other to come to their own conclusions. But every now and then, Cam glanced at Tabernacle imploringly, and after a while, the custodian took note.

'I heard everything that man out there said about you,' said Tabernacle. 'About what you're dealing with and what you've been through. This must feel like a lifeline of sorts.'

Cam hated it when people assumed they knew where his head was at. But it had been laid bare so many times this evening already, once more couldn't hurt him. 'I'm not asking you to do anything,' he said. 'Not physical, not out there, just turn a blind eye and give me a bit of local know-how. Can you do that for me?'

Tabernacle waited a couple of moments before responding, as if sizing up not just the man sat opposite him, but his chances of success too. Cam held his gaze, his jaw set.

'All right,' said Tabernacle eventually.

'Thank you.' Cam then smiled. 'So … is Feather House still standing?' Since the abandoned home had come up, Cam had been unable to stop wondering if any clues had been left there too.

Tabernacle sighed with resignation. 'Yes. It's got a big fence around it though, watched by a security firm.'

That sounded troublesome to Cam, but when Tabernacle saw his disappointment, he spoke again. 'But it was a local security firm, and it couldn't survive all that COVID. It went bust a while back. You look like you can climb a fence.'

Cam brightened. It was on. 'You said it's not far away. Would you be able to point me in the right direction?'

Tabernacle shook his head in admonishment, but at last smiled himself. 'I will, but you didn't get it from me.'

24

It turned out that the only real way to get to the building known as Brindley Hall was via yet more water – or at least the outer edges of a small private lake. Fifteen minutes' drive from Hickling Broad, through roads so dark tonight it felt like they would go on forever. Cam's van had already nearly rendered a handful of pheasants two-dimensional. Once he'd parked in a tractor turning and hopped out, Nala on his heels, he took out his phone and used it to navigate through some of the most sprawling undergrowth he'd ever come across.

The fence appeared as promised, partially swallowed by the hungry foliage. A sign on it read MacReady Security Solutions, and Cam wondered what they were up to now. He put a hand on it, half-expecting sirens to go off or that he'd be run through by ten thousand volts, but nothing happened. Tabernacle had suggested he might climb it, but Cam had brought wire cutters from the depths of his van. As he snipped clear a small opening, he wondered who on earth had arranged for this to be set up in the first place. Either way, he and Nala were soon through, and he'd angle that query to the eager minds of Gupta and Ferris.

As they clomped through the brush, Cam started to hear monkeys. Whooping and bellowing. Mating cries, or excitement, or just for the hell of it. It was other-worldly and intimidating, and if it weren't for the fact that Tabernacle had tipped Cam off that this would happen, he would be totally disturbed. The simple explanation was that Brindley Hall was not too far away from Thrigby Hall Wildlife Park and its various primate residents. That didn't completely erase the unease though, especially as what he guessed was a gibbon's plaintive howls carried across the pool towards him, in yet more near-infinite blackness.

Nala again, was absolutely delighted to be on an adventure with her master. She trotted ahead of him through the undergrowth, every now and then popping her head up to see if he was following, as he tramped around an overgrown lake in the middle of an even more overgrown garden.

'Yes, yes. I'm right behind you'.

Across the moonlit water, some fifty metres away, sat a house in side profile. Dark windows watched him as he walked. It was a husk, empty and bereft of human life, but he felt he couldn't escape its gaze. It gave him the creeps.

But he would not be perturbed. Whether this place had answers or not he wouldn't know until he entered and gave the house a thorough search – and he'd come too far to turn back now. The ferns licked and gripped the hem of his dryrobe and soaked his calves, and all the while he kept watch on the darkness on the other side of the water, scanning for movement.

The building itself was, as an outdated expression might have it, a pile. Choked with plant life, it looked as if it was being sucked back into the forest. It had two storeys, and huge windows in varying states of disrepair on every side, belying vast rooms and a once elite standard of living. Cam wasn't sure he'd ever set foot in such a house in his life. He remembered there was a modest palace in Afghanistan that carried a similar level of scale and opulence, but never anything so close to home.

As he ventured around the far end of the lake, tight to a deep band of forest he could see no further than a couple of metres into, Nala appeared on a rise ahead of him and barked. She was noticeably higher up than Cam was. He looked through the vegetation around his ankles and sure enough, his wet shoes hit thick stone steps. They were covered almost completely by ferns and decay, but to the touch, rock solid.

With great care, he navigated his way up to join Nala on the pathway towards Brindley Hall itself. He turned for one last look at the lake. The moon glimmered on the still surface. He couldn't help wondering what it would be like to dive in.

As Cam looked at the glassy surface, he took out his phone, and dialled the number he'd saved as soon as he received it. It was answered after only a couple of rings.

'You do know what time it is?' came the weary voice of DS Rogers.

'Thought I'd check in while I had a minute,' said Cam. 'Sorry if I disturbed you. I wanted to keep you on top of things.'

'I know you're a social misfit, Killick, but do you have any idea what time it is? I mean it.'

Cam didn't. 'No idea. Listen, I found something at the bottom of Hickling. A kid's toy dog. It could be Hannah Brindley's – it was only a matter of metres from where I found the car.'

He heard a male voice murmuring, then Rogers hissing the word *twat*. There was rustling, then Rogers' voice took on an echo. 'Go on.'

'Another interested party came to see me. Someone new. An older man. I didn't get a good look at him. I'm now out at Brindley Hall, seeing if there's anything to find.'

Rogers swore under her breath. 'I didn't hear that,' she said. 'You've got to be careful there, Cam. Don't leave any evidence you've been. If my superiors find out you've been crusading, they'll come down on you heavily.'

'I'll be careful. What's happening your way?' He had no idea whether Rogers would answer that question, so he was delighted when she did. It meant, more than anything, that he'd gained her trust, or some modicum of it.

'Listen, you never heard me say this, but you might have been right about the police.' Her voice was loaded with sarcasm. 'And I may or may not have enjoyed a couple of additional glasses of wine going over the full case documentation. The *actual* full case documentation. I managed to get the entirety of the case folder copied – took me a very sweaty forty minutes and a full change of ink. But that's not the only thing, Cam. You won't believe it – it's different to the official one I had access to. When the chief took it from me to close the case, he put all sorts back into it. It's almost like all this time, there were two separate case files.'

The subterfuge was deeply disturbing, but aside from that, this was good news. Having all the Brindley case information to hand gave Rogers autonomy from the station.

'Nice work,' Cam said.

'And I found something interesting,' she said.

Cam held still and stared at the water. 'Go on.'

'Amongst the new stuff, was something I've never seen before. The night they were last seen, the party at the mayor's house? I've got a guest list.'

The picture of the Brindleys on the steps – the image of the man, half-hidden in shadow who had drawn Tommy's eye – burst into Cam's mind. 'Do you, now?'

'In the file was a statement taken from a Mrs Gillian Reynolds – Mayor Reynolds' wife. Investigating officers visited them three weeks after the party, when the family had first been reported missing.'

Cam heard the urgency in her speech. 'And?'

'Very simple statement, the whole thing seemed to be handled with kid gloves, given who they were interviewing. But she did offer a list of people that had come that night.'

'That's great. Any names pop out?'

'Not yet,' Rogers said. 'But it's a who's who of local eighties heavyweights. I'll get you a copy when I can. I'm going to give it some thought.'

'Me too,' said Cam. 'Anything else?'

'No, unless you want to hear about the car park ticket fraud case the higher-ups have put me on?'

'Nah, you're all right.' They agreed to keep in touch, and Cam thanked her and clicked off.

He flicked across to the WhatsApp group Gupta and Ferris had made, which contained just the three of them. Ferris had insisted on calling it WE WANT TO BELIEVE, with a picture of a UFO as its avatar. After Rogers' admonishments, he decided not to call and typed out a text.

Anything on Belvedere yet?

He lowered the phone and took in his surroundings once more. Turning back to the building, Cam saw a stone path drawn around its base, tight to the filthy stone walls covered in lichen, vines and all manner of floral bric-a-brac. Even for a man in Cam's physical condition, travelling the path wasn't easy, but Nala showed him the safest way, her instinct for sure footing as strong as ever. The walk gave him a sense of the property's dimensions. It really was a mansion in every sense, surrounded on each side by extensive, once-landscaped examples of topiary, lawns and carefully selected plants, the latter of which stood outsized and distended like sore agricultural thumbs.

In the moonlight, all of this flora looked black. It was only the eaves and gables of Brindley Hall that were unmarked and unravaged by the night's onyx grip, the vines unable to reach quite so high. The windows themselves looked vacant, like the dull stare of a huge doll.

He reached the far corner of the house and found what appeared to be the front entrance.

Wading through grass that came up to his waist, Cam saw a grand, columned porch raised before the front door. As he got closer, he noticed that the grass had not been able to penetrate the porch's marble, and desiccated leaves covered the once-ornate flooring.

But it was at the door that Cam's heart stuck in his throat and his knees threatened to wobble. On any other night, the sight wouldn't have affected him like this, but after what he'd found on the bottom of Hickling Broad, finding four pairs of wellington boots, lined up in size order next to the front door, was almost too much to bear. It looked like the owners would be coming out any moment, ready for another day in the green embrace of the Norfolk countryside. He let his torchlight illuminate

them fully. Four wellies, two adult pairs, and beside them
two children's pairs, the larger; blue and covered in rockets,
the smaller; pink with faded ponies on the side.

Use it Cam, he told himself.

His stomach lurched at the thought that the rest of the
building would be exactly the same as it had been left.
Maybe a kettle still on the hob, with a couple of mugs or
a teapot, bags at the ready.

His phone chirped. A reply from the *Norfolk Unexplained*
team. As he opened the app, he saw there'd been a couple
of messages.

> **Gupta**
> French investment company. Registered
> November 1987. Owns all sorts of land
> and property across UK and France.
> Not massive but big enough.

> **Ferris**
> The only things they own
> in Norfolk are that strip
> alongside Hickling, and a
> property over in Thrigby.

> **Gupta**
> Yeah. A place called Feather House.

> **Ferris**
> We kept our mouths shut
> at the press conference
> as requested.

Feather House. The name echoed a chime in Cam's
head. That was exactly where he was standing. Tabernacle
said so – it was the building's original name. Maybe it
was changed back officially after the disappearance of

154

the Brindleys? Maybe it had never had an official name change at all?

But there was no coincidence in it. There couldn't be. Belvedere owning the last resting place of the Brindley car *and* the abandoned Brindley home?

Cam hadn't even needed to ask those journo-podcasting-conspiracy-theorists about the fence after all. They'd already answered it. Belvedere, again.

Keep looking into Belvedere, he typed. *And thank you.*

The building in front of him took on even more weight and importance. Cam tried the front door. It was glass-panelled with frosted panes and held fast against his weight. The panes rattled. But a couple of well-placed barges from the meat of his shoulder (the one that wasn't bruised) and he was in. Brindley Hall, and all its secrets, yawned at him through the swinging front door.

He took one last look around the overgrown front garden and the drive. There was nothing and nobody. With a deep breath he didn't mean to take, he stepped inside.

25

The sun came up around half seven, just as Cam was entering the final throes of his search. Now down to the last couple of rooms, he'd been up for some twenty-five hours, but carried no signs of tiredness. A control held him, which was all the more amazing given the length of time it had been since his last chemical cocktail. He could've gone home hours ago, of course, come back today to carry on the job, but he felt that if he paused his urgency, momentum would go with it.

He also had to admit that he liked the feeling of possible discovery. It was both fresh and a welcome return at the same time.

Despite himself, Cam actually found the house quite scary. Haunting, in that, just as he expected, it had been abandoned. It was like a normal day had passed, and the people inside had just been vaporised, dusted into the heavens. He kept expecting to see things out of the corner of his eye, and more than once let his mind wander so far he had to check again to make sure he really was alone.

It was painful, at times *very* painful, sifting through the last moments of a family who had abruptly disappeared. He saw echoes of them laid bare in every corner of the house.

Tommy's bedroom revealed a long-standing obsession with boats. Homemade art projects hung everywhere, that had graduated from infantile blunt shapes in paintings to dedicated model-making with high-end kits.

The little girl's room, Hannah, betrayed a deep love of all things animal, a cream and purple safe haven of a seven-year-old's hopes and dreams.

It gave him a profound ache, just to stand in those rooms.

He checked on Nala before heading into the down-stairs office, the room he had deliberately picked to attack in daylight. The dog was lying where she had been for some hours now, asleep by the kitchen Aga, huddled on a blanket that had been left there on that fateful, final day. Sensing his presence, she looked up at him with an expression that seem to say, *yes?* He smiled at her, glad she was with him. Trawling through this empty edifice all night was an unsettling task.

As Cam crossed the hall, avoiding the piles of leaves that had got in through a shattered window in one of the front bays, he braced himself to enter the world of the parents.

He'd seen roughly what they were about in the other rooms in the house – particularly the bedroom, a garish cavern of absurdly dense wallpaper and a four-poster bed on an elevated platform. Then there had been the living room – or perhaps these people called it a drawing room? – which housed a huge, boxy television that the whole family could've had dinner in if only its innards were removed.

A glance through their domains quickly revealed their tastes. Freddie Brindley was into fishing, expensive watches and tailored shoes. Maud Brindley was into photography, books, horses and music – with the most expensive ward-robe he'd ever seen. They seemed the typical well-to-do country couple, but there were so many blanks that needed filling in, and he felt sure that myths of history had for so long skewed the real story.

As soon as he walked into the downstairs office, Cam realised that another window had been shattered somewhere, and, because the room was so small compared to the others, the entire office was dusted in dirt and leaves. He stood on the threshold, taking it all in, and trying to commit it to memory.

It was decorated in a deeply textured black wallpaper, torn in many places in long strips. To the immediate left of the door was a bookcase still full of weighty tomes, which at a glance all bore titles to do with accountancy, investments and money management. The word *wealth* featured on what he guessed could be about twenty of those spines. He knew that Freddie was involved in the world of finance and city banking, travelling regularly to London and back again. These books affirmed that suggestion, but clarified the man's true calling, suggesting him to be somewhat of a personal wealth manager. Who for, nobody had ever said. Cam hoped such answers would be in this very room.

On a desk in the middle were two items of real interest. A vintage Apple Macintosh, possibly the very first model of its kind, and on top of that, sat proudly like a jaunty hat, a bird's nest, long abandoned, its walls and shape defined by an assortment of small twigs and those missing strips of wallpaper.

Behind the desk was a window made up of rows of small panes, one of which was missing, presumably where the opportunistic homemaker had come through. The right-hand wall housed an old, rusted filing cabinet, three drawers high, and next to it a display of vintage golf clubs. They started with old wooden models on the left-hand side before taking more modern shapes – well, up to the mid-eighties at least. It fit the bill, the finance prince heading to the country and dabbling in the expensive end of his outdoorsy hobbies.

Above all this was a blank wall – too blank, Cam thought.

He crossed the room, avoiding as much of the in-blown detritus as he could, and examined the wall. The light was fine with the dawn glare through the window, but an instinct made him click on his torch. Across the wall's surface were a series of small, lined shadows, like spikes. They swayed and warped as he swung the light along them.

Nails.

Pictures must have hung on that wall. All gone. All quite small, judging by the spacing of the metalwork. No bigger than eight by ten inches. Now, if this place really had been abandoned exactly as it was on their final day, why had Freddie taken all these pictures down?

And where were they now? He hadn't seen a pile of photographs anywhere, nor was there a similar photo wall in any of the other rooms, which would suggest they had merely been moved. So where would you store them? He hadn't seen a garage on his brief tour of the outskirts of the property, but maybe there was an outbuilding he'd missed, buried under the encroaching forest. Maybe the attic? He'd have to go back and check.

From the wall, he moved along to the filing cabinet and pulled open the top drawer. He knew, as soon as he yanked the handle and felt no resistance, that it was going to be empty. True enough, it was – save for a few empty folders and unused labels lying at the bottom. He quickly checked them – all blank. Spares. The real folders had gone.

One part of Cam had been expecting all manner of printouts, reports, forms he could go through over the coming days to try to find out if Freddie Brindley had done anything dodgy enough to get himself in trouble, like embezzling funds. But no.

Unlike the rest of the house, which lay relatively undisturbed, the office had been cleaned out.

There was, however, one stone still unturned. The computer.

He'd checked the light switches when he entered the house and, obviously, nothing illuminated – but now he checked the one on the wall for completion's sake. Nothing. He doubted he'd be able to see what was on the screen anyway through its impressionist spatter of bird shit. He'd have to get that computer out of here, somewhere he could take a better look at it or get someone to rip the hard drive. There was a possible bank of information just sitting there, and it would be wrong of him to overlook it.

And then, he heard Nala's growl.

Cam's head snapped up.

She never did that. Not unless…

He threw himself at the computer, bird shit be damned, ripping out ancient cables and pulling the entire unit into his grasp, sending a confetti of twigs and wallpaper flying. Carrying it to the door, he met Nala coming the other way.

'Someone here?' he asked in a whisper, as they darted in tandem back into the hall. Cam hung close to the walls as he approached the front windows.

He felt completely naked holding the boxy computer unit, and not a weapon.

The glass in the bay windows either side of the front door was caked in a film of grime, but he could see through it well enough – to spy three men tramping through the grass, their steps high and long to avoid the reaching blades.

26

Three on one. They were coming up the grass, quick and heavy-looking, scoping out the property with thick, swivelling necks. This time, in his fight or flight calculations, which only took Cam a fraction of a second, the latter emerged the stronger option of success.

'Nala,' he hissed, 'let's go, *now*.'

And he ran, holding the computer. Nala was suddenly ahead of him, both of them angling for the kitchen and the back door he had located during his search.

He cursed himself for not trying to re-lock the front door after they'd entered, and even worse, he found the back door was shut fast. He barged it twice, but it was no good. The windows over the sink, while mucky and faded, were all largely intact too. Nothing he could get through without unleashing an unholy racket.

'Come on, Nala,' he said as he ran back out of the kitchen to the hall and poked his head around the door frame. The glass in the front door was empty of shapes, but he knew they were only seconds away. 'Upstairs,' he said, and Nala darted up along the decaying banisters, Cam following two at a time behind.

They hit the landing and Nala turned to wait for instruction. There were voices on the porch downstairs. The sudden rise in tension threatened to throw away all his composure, all that calm he'd carefully harvested, and the dogs of PTSD were abruptly straining at their leashes. Everything was a split second from unravelling.

Hold it together, hold it to-fucking-gether.

Why had these men come *now?* Brindley Hall had been sat here for forty years, undisturbed. What was it about the discovery of the car that had kicked them into action after all this time? What was it they were looking for? Had they followed him? Cam hadn't seen anybody either, but still, it was heavily signposted that the site was watched.

Either way, he didn't fancy his chances of escaping the place with an entire eighties computer in tow.

'Creepy,' said a voice downstairs.

They were in.

Cam looked at Nala and gave the tiniest *shush* for all the good that would do. Pins and needles swarmed his back.

Hold it together. They might not even know you're here.

He listened, still as he could be, as three distinct sets of footsteps made their way onto the tile of the hallway. A voice parched by age and inflected with weariness echoed through the building.

'All right, gents, let's get this place turned over quick as we can. Find the photographs, and I'll buy you lunch.'

Cam stood on the upstairs landing, utterly frozen. The voice. He recognised it. The man from the night before, in the trees. He clearly wasn't one for giving up.

But photographs? Is that what this whole thing was about? Some pictures?

Pictures. The row of nails in the wall downstairs.

The pictures clearly missing from the wall in Freddie's office.

Holy *hell*, thought Cam, electrified, as the dots connected.

But there was no time to think of where they'd been stashed now – he had to get himself hidden, and fast, if the men were going to start turning the house over. Only after that could he look for those pictures himself, and make sure he found them first.

Cam tried to think of hiding places on the top floor. The massive armoire wardrobe in the master suite would be the first place anyone would look. The linen closet was the same. And even if he could get into the loft through the tiny hatch overhead, he'd never manage it with a dog and a heavy Apple computer. And then an idea hit him that was so absurd, it had to work. He'd seen it earlier. Thought you could fit a whole person in it.

Wordlessly, although Nala got the message and followed, he tiptoed as quick as he could into Hannah Brindley's bedroom. In the corner was an antique behemoth of a dollhouse, with one hinged gable end you could open. He pulled it open, saw the small space inside. It would be a squeeze, but what the fuck other chance did he have? He clambered in with the computer and the dog.

It was very narrow inside, designed for a child to play in the central column of the house, surrounded by rooms on either side. Only problem was, once he had wedged his backside between the two halves of the house, the windows, themselves immaculate miniatures, clearly betrayed what was beyond the inside of the tiny rooms. *Himself.* He pulled off his dryrobe from the hood and blocked them from the inside, praying that would be enough.

Fully wedged in now, he pulled Nala close, stroking her chin and staring into her eyes imploringly. Nala stared back at him, doing a very good job of suggesting she had got the message. *Silence.*

Cam's next battle, the one that was growing in prominence with every hushed breath, was with nerves.

If there was ever a time for anxiety to run rampant, it was now.

He wanted to scream the house down, shout till his lungs bled. And with the pressure on him so high, all he could see in his head was bloodshed. The old injuries of colleagues long since fallen, the spatter of his own bullets finding their target. The grim aftermath of those moments, wiping off the claret both physically and mentally. In high tensile situations, this unwanted portfolio paraded in front of his eyes. Usually going underwater or choking down a higher dose of his pharmaceutical concoction would do to clear it – but Cam had neither option to hand.

It was just him, Nala and hope. A battle of wits and nerve, both of which had deserted him in recent years.

Cam sat in the cold grip of the dollhouse as beyond and below, the men tore Brindley Hall in half. Shattering and crashing rang from every room, footsteps pounded this way and that. It was less of a subtle search than a demolition job by hand.

By finding the car, he'd set off an urgent chain of events. Seemingly the Brindley mystery was of no importance when it was dormant, but now the car had been found, old secrets had resurfaced with it. And a lot of it, apparently, centred on some photographs – photographs that were assumed lost with the Brindleys – but when they weren't discovered in the car, now needed to be urgently recovered.

Whenever the noises got past a certain decibel level, Nala looked up at him. He held her gaze, watching the worry glint in her eyes. But she never made a sound. He knew, however, that the time was coming when the thugs would reach the little girl's bedroom, and sure enough, with a smash of the door and the immediate flipping of what sounded like the bed, they were in.

Two distinct sets of footsteps hurried all around them, their owners wordlessly breaking the room to pieces. Nala started to squirm as floorboards shook. Cam carefully held her muzzle and put his forehead to hers.

He expected discovery any second. With sudden violence, the dollhouse was yanked and one of the internal upstairs floors of the toy dug into Cam's back, lodging between two notches in his spine. He wanted to scream, but instead bit his lip so hard he tasted blood. The dollhouse was shoved the other way, crushing into his shins. The men didn't realise you could open it, so were trying to pull it apart with sheer force. Nala tried to make a break for it, but he held her tight. He wanted to shout, just to break the tension, but jammed his teeth together instead, biting the fear back down his throat.

'Spoiled brats, this thing is sturdier than the house I grew up in,' one of the thugs spat, and kicked the wall of the dollhouse like an impotent exclamation mark.

It stopped as abruptly as it had started. They clearly thought the thing was just a toy. Nothing more than a heavy, fixed, rich kids' plaything. Nala settled back down as they listened to the men get to work on the wardrobes. They heard clothes hangers crash onto the floor and the occasional tinkle of split glass, then, with a loud 'Fuck it', they left.

Cam didn't dare breathe a sigh of relief for a full five minutes.

27

Fifteen more minutes passed while the sweat cooled on Cam's skin, until loud steps down the stairs rang out. They were accompanied by a bellowed 'Upstairs is clear', followed shortly by a question: 'Any luck down here?'

'No, nothing here either,' came the reply.

For all their crashing about and bluster, they hadn't found a thing.

Cam almost smiled to himself. But he wasn't out yet.

He did however decide it was time to get out of the dollhouse, and ever so gingerly, he parted the front and back walls to peek out. The coast was mercifully clear – but the room looked post-bomb strike.

Everything that wasn't glued down was broken and upended, and it saddened Cam no end.

That little girl, missing for almost forty years … now her precious things were destroyed because of some grown-ups making bad decisions.

He carried Nala onto the landing and they listened at the top of the stairs as the men reconvened in the echoing hallway.

'So we've got nothing. Nothing to take back at all.' This was the voice of the apparent leader – the one who'd waited for him to come out of Hickling Broad last night.

'Just a load of dusty old crap.'

A new voice. But something about it felt familiar to Cam too.

'I reckon there's nothing left to find now.'

'So what are we going to do?'

'I guess we go and see the diver,' said the man from the night before.

The words hit like an anvil strike in Cam's chest.

Cam had become a serious shit magnet, and now it seemed that Haven Cottage was no longer a haven at all.

The men kept chuntering to each other as they left the property, and Cam was able finally to breathe easy. Well, easier, at least.

He wandered through the rubble of their search and made his way into the master bedroom. The destruction was even worse in here – not so much a bomb as a meteor strike. The wardrobes were now in pieces, a shattered skeleton of wood on the floor, the thrown clothes, their splayed cotton innards.

He crept across the debris, careful not to step on any glass from the ornate chandelier that had been pulled down, presumably more out of frustration than out of any serious expectation that it was hiding lost photographs.

As he watched the men beat their way back through the overgrown lawn, he wondered what made these missing photographs so important – and whether they'd ever been in the house at all.

Would photographs of such obvious concern even be displayed on a wall? But then again, he thought, looking at the carnage of opulence he was standing in, he had no idea how people of this social standing behaved. The whole place had been a garish monument to Freddie Brindley's success, with many features Cam would never dream of having in his own home, no matter how much money was in his bank account. Glass statues of distended naked bodies that could be high art for all he knew. A large painting of a white tiger driving a Ferrari. A portrait – not of the whole family, but of Freddie Brindley himself.

Outside, one of the men slipped in the grass and went down face first, losing himself fully to the sea of green. Cam would have laughed if the whole thing wasn't so damn serious. As the man righted himself, Cam caught a clear look at his face. Without question, it was the man from the woods by Hickling Broad.

He was older than the others. Stocky. Wearing a thick dark coat that hung down somewhere into the overflowing tide of grass. His face was thickened by the wrinkled jowls of extremely prosperous living, and his brown hair fell in a neat side parting on a wide bowling ball of a head.

Cam heard the expletives clearly through the old glass, and listened as the man berated his chuckling colleagues. One of the other men turned round and smiled darkly through a thick black beard.

No, thought Cam – followed by *of course*. He looked again at the two other men, walking away, and saw that one had a pronounced white bandage on his cheek.

It was the thugs from a couple of nights back – well, the two that could still walk; the leader and Little King Henry with the fried face. They carried themselves like old-school muscle, all bunched shoulders, jagged elbows and long strides.

There weren't two parties after all – they were all in on this together.

Once they'd gone all the way down the drive, Cam finally turned to Nala and stroked behind her ears. 'Good job, you,' he said. 'That was tight.'

He checked his watch. Ten in the morning. Their search had taken about two hours. Not their first rodeo, to toss a place of this size with such abandon and speed.

The day had broken into a pleasant morning, with some unseasonal sunlight glinting off the lake. The water looked biting and murky, small waves cresting with a lip of white on the surface, caused by the breeze that seemed ever-present around here.

The water.

It hit Cam like a truck.

The only place they hadn't searched.

Cam thought fast – did he have a spare tank in his van? He had one empty one, he knew that much. But all his kit was there. Even if there was only enough air in one of his other tanks for fifteen minutes, it was worth it.

28

Pulling on a cold, soaking wetsuit was one of the worst parts of a professional diver's job – but doing it after being awake for more than a full day rendered the task even more uncomfortable.

Cam had checked through the four tanks in his van and found one with about half an hour's worth left. That was better than he'd hoped for.

He had stashed the old computer in the van, wrapped in one of the dog blankets, and stowed it under the shelves out of sight. Then he took his kit back through the woods to the water's edge, suited up under Nala's watchful eye, and carefully walked into the lake next to Brindley Hall. The water was frigid – what did he expect? – but the fact that he was already in a cold wetsuit meant the temperature didn't even register as he strode in.

This was, he conceded, a stupid idea.

He knew nothing about this water. He didn't know how deep it was, what underwater obstacles there might be, or really, what he was looking for. More stupid once again, was the fact he was diving alone. The number of common-sense diving rules he'd broken in the last few days was too many to count. But he felt that self-imposed duty, and Hannah Brindley's pleading gaze through the mists of history, push him forward.

With every footstep, he tested his footing, knowing that any mistakes he made wouldn't just slow him down, they might kill him. Earlier on in his diving career, thoughts like this might have been dismissed with bravado. These days, he knew that thinking about the worst possibilities was what kept him alive.

He was only up to his chest now, but every footstep felt like he was charging slowly through vines. Ordinarily, ornamental lakes such as this one would be regularly dredged, the banks pruned, the water frequently tested for levels of acidity and sediment. Those obstacles littering his route into the pond were things that would usually have been fished out long ago. Downed branches, dead leaves, old pondweed and the roots of lily pad systems. He turned and gave Nala one last look, then lowered his head under the water. After the last however many fraught hours, the cool squeeze was blissful, and the knots in Cam's neck instantly eased.

He immediately sank to his haunches and then forward to lie on his chest. The water was as murky as he'd ever seen it in Norfolk, the colour of three-day-old hot chocolate. The only thing he could do was, like a bloodhound following an aniseed trail, stick his nose to the deck and follow it hand over hand. If he encountered a downed tree limb, he could end up with a stuck tank – or worse, a stuck torso – which would pin him in place until both the tank and his own lungs gave way and left him just another secret lost to Brindley Hall.

Cam had decided a long time ago, despite the risks of his occupation, that drowning wasn't the way he wanted to go.

He traced the bottom of the lake as it dipped gradually deeper. The lake was a hundred metres long, and maybe seventy metres wide at its broadest point, and experience told him it couldn't possibly be very deep, but caution was the friend that kept him alive. To that end, he considered every move carefully.

The bottom of the lake was very different to the silty base of Hickling Broad. Here it was more of a mulch, a pile of sudden desiccation that looked like drains and gutters had been emptied into it. If anything had been down here for forty years, it would almost certainly be completely buried by now under all this filth and decomposing floral matter.

To check his watch for readings, Cam had to bring his entire wrist right up to his eyes and illuminate the dial with his other hand. He did so now and saw that he had twenty minutes left underwater.

His intention was to focus on the bankside water closest to the house, following the logic that if you were throwing something out to sink in here, you would do so at the nearest point between the house and the water. It was a game of probabilities, but he found that a lot of the time, human behaviour followed such patterns. He remembered from earlier that morning that you could see the lake out of Freddie's office window – to get rid of something, you only had to glance out the window for inspiration of where to stick it.

When he reached his proposed fifteen metre distance from the bank and hadn't found anything, he span in place to face the bank again, and crab-walked a metre to his right before crawling back. The return leg was full of similar underwater features, and as soon as his head broke the surface, he span again and crab-walked left this time, dragging himself along back out towards the centre of the lake.

It was after two more repetitions and five minutes of air that he found something.

A plastic sack.

He would've missed it if it weren't for the distinct bulge protruding from the bottom. It was the same silty colour as the rest of the mud, but the shape of it – bulbous and angular – made him brush at some of the wet mud to reveal an entire sack. He tested the weight by gripping the knot and gently lifting. It was heavy enough, but he could lift it, releasing a cloud of thick sediment as he did so. He put a hand underneath it and took its weight. The last thing he needed was the bag to split and the contents to spill into the murk. But as his hands touched it, he felt that whatever was inside the bag was jagged and movable, with sharp corners. Excitement galloped at what could be inside, hoping his deductions were right.

Cam carefully held the sack in his arms as he stood and marched back up to the bank, spitting out his regulator as his face broke the surface.

'We might've been lucky here, girl,' he said to Nala, as he climbed over the reeds and placed the bag onto the stone path. In the cold sunlight the mud looked almost black and chunky, but it was full of partially decomposed leaves that brushed away easily with a shake of the bag. It was a grey rubble sack, made of industrial strength plastic. The top had been folded over and stapled shut. Hurriedly, Cam took off his mask and started to pick at the staples. It had been fastened tight, and it took him a while to undo enough to get a look inside. At last, he managed to part the opening of the bag and peer inside.

'Oh, yes. Jackpot'.

Poking his hand in, with a scrape and a tinkle of something loose and metal, he pulled out a photo frame and held it out for inspection. The frame was damaged at the corner, and water leakage had entered both the bag and the frame's contents. The photograph behind the small pane of glass was running and faded at the corners, colours and ink whirling into each other in a watercolour mess – but to his amazement the subject at the centre of the image was clear enough to see.

Freddie Brindley was in the middle of the frame, shaking hands with another man. They were standing on the steps of what look like a nightclub or show venue, the name 'Birds Nest' in neon strips framed by those dressing room mirror lightbulbs. They were both dressed in finery, with faces that said they were in the grip of a damn good time.

It was a window into the life of a man Cam had only known in death. Freddie looked like he had the world at his feet. The other man had the paunch of the well-to-do, the expensive suit and the crooked, smug smile of someone born for moments like these. The face rang a bell in the back of Cam's head, but the tune was a mystery. Nevertheless, more fragments about the Brindley case were being revealed at last, and it gave Cam a determined buoyancy. He didn't know who the people in the pictures were, but they were obviously important – not just to Freddie Brindley, but to the thugs on their tail too.

Placing this first one on the grass, the grey sky above shimmering in the glass, he took another look in the bag. It was full of similar framed photos – maybe twenty of them.

What had he found here? What did these images mean?

He looked down the drive. The men hadn't reappeared, but he couldn't risk them coming back and finding him

174

here with the photographs they'd ripped the house up for. He had to get these out of here and spread them out for proper inspection. His excitement was rising again. He felt sure the answers were closer than they had been before.

'I don't think we can go home, girl, or at least not yet. We need to find a doggie hotel for a couple of days.'

Nala licked his hand and snuffed back dismissively. 'I know, I know I need a shower too.'

He stood, picked up the bag and walked through the grass towards his van – to find somewhere he could go through all this evidence quietly, discreetly and above all, safely.

29

With the sack of photo frames safely stored in the back of his van alongside the computer, Cam began the drive back towards civilisation, with a sense of satisfaction of a job well done. However, with every passing turn, this soon gave way to uncertainty.

Where to go now?

The men who had turned Brindley Hall upside down had said the next port of call would be 'the diver'. Cam, himself. He knew from experience that they interrogated like they searched. Cam didn't want to be there for round two.

There were all sorts of places he could lie low. He could even sleep in the van if he wanted to. But his van itself was a marker, and if those men knew what he drove, it made him recognisable in an instant.

Wherever he parked up, it would have to be out of sight.

He also needed amenities. He hadn't eaten in hours and could do with being in hitting distance of a pharmacy in case he needed to get back on his meds urgently. He was amazed he'd made it this far without having an attack of some kind. On top of this, he'd been awake for almost twenty-eight hours, with two dives in that time.

He needed a shower, food and rest.

He needed somewhere he would feel comfortable enough to get those things, without provoking his anxiety into reacting.

As he drove, Cam thought of the places where he had truly felt at ease while living down here in Norfolk. This list was short, but after a few moments he remembered one spot he'd enjoyed. A place that, even while he was in the starting stages of the breakdown that came to define the years since, he'd felt respite.

He angled the van on a course along the A47 to Wroxham, reaching for his phone as he did so, to plug it into the cigarette charger. When he had first come to Norfolk, as part of the SBS diving and recovery unit, it was to fish a helicopter out of the river Bure in front of a pub called the Penny Black, which had been the unlikely setting for a gang related shootout. How the helicopter had ended up in the water, he never found out, although the bodies recovered showed evidence of one hell of a scrap.

When they were on jobs, they usually had digs provided – and for this case those digs were in Wroxham, at the imaginatively monikered Hotel Wroxham. It had been quiet, clean, full of good food and drink, with comfortable rooms that overlooked the water. It also had a car park behind the building, out of sight of the main road – perfect for his van. Plus, Wroxham itself had an array of shops and a department store. He was desperate for a change of clothes. Cam seemed to recall, as the cherry on the cake, that the hotel was dog-friendly.

In short, it would be perfect.

It was about a half an hour drive away, but that would give him time to book in advance; a necessity because he didn't want to show up at the front desk looking like this and for them to have an excuse to say, 'no room at the inn'. As soon as his phone had enough charge, he pulled over into a layby and went on Booking.com.

After the ups and downs of the last couple of days, Wroxham felt like another planet. People were going about their business as usual, paying no heed to the worse-for-wear stranger with the small dog who had wandered into their midst.

But why would they? It was the same when he was in the military. Whatever he did on foreign shores, in combat situations riddled with bullets and blood, it was always so the people back home could go about their lives with freedom. And if ignorance of their protectors was part of the deal, he'd always been cool with that.

Cam parked his van in the car park behind Hotel Wroxham and walked the short hop past the post office and the fishing tackle shop to Roys department store. Roys stores were split by a road right through the middle – with half on one side, half on the other. The segment on the other side of the street housed the pharmacy, giftware and the more high-end labelled goods. The building that Cam had walked into was the food hall, which also housed a McDonald's and the more fiscally conscious clothing choices.

He collected a few looks on the way in thanks to his filthy face, dryrobe and wet shoes so, head down, walked straight over to the racks of men's clothing. He grabbed items without much thought, the first pinpricks of emotional discomfort crackling in his belly. A pair of jeans and a couple of thick corded fisherman's jumpers. A packet of underwear, a packet of socks and a five pack of basic T-shirts. That was all he needed – he had spare trainers in the car, and his dryrobe would act as a coat.

He took the pile to the checkout, and it was at this point that the accumulated adrenaline finally ebbed out of his system – only to be replaced by something else. As the buzz left his veins one way, an angry tingle went the other. It started in his head, underneath his hair. It cast along his cheekbones, down the tendons and cords of his neck, through his shoulders and along his biceps to his forearms. And that was where they began to burn and itch, fire and ice and lice, all mixed together.

Standing still was driving him mad. There were six people in the line in front of him. Everyone was elderly, and he wished they'd get a bloody move on. He immediately chastised himself for the thought – but he couldn't help it. He was beginning to feel desperate.

Get a move on.

Hurry the fuck up.

Sweat popped on Cam's brow and soon a trickle pumped down his forehead, collecting mud as it went, getting darker as it reached the tip of his nose. His left leg started to tremor, his foot began to tap. He knew he looked like a dirty picture of impatience, but there was nothing he could do.

He started to breathe carefully to ward off the panic attack. *In for three, hold for five, out for eight.* But all that did was draw looks, adding to his anxiety.

He debated running across the road to the pharmacy to get an emergency supply of meds. But he was torn. Notwithstanding how he was feeling now, he liked how on edge he had been for the last day or so. He'd managed to hold back these attacks with proactivity and productivity, with the drive of obsession pulling his attention elsewhere. And it had been *working*. He didn't want to take a backward step now. He'd been rediscovering his own powers of control, hour by hour, and he didn't want to undo it.

Suddenly, Cam felt a hand land onto his own clammy forearm. He jumped, startled, and looked down to find an elderly lady with a tartan push-trolley and a kind expression. She had to have been all of ninety years old, and her thumb traced a juddering circle on his forearm.

'Calm down, love,' she said. 'Better to be five minutes late in this life, than five minutes early in the next.'

He put his own quivering hand on hers and squeezed. 'Thank you,' he said.

They stayed that way until he got to the front of the queue, hand-in-hand, while his panic attack passed. She seemed to know what he needed, the kind of innate knowledge only experience and a love for the good in people could grant.

When he got to the front, Cam asked if she had anything to buy. The woman held out a pair of child's wellies. The sight of more kids' wellies took him back to Brindley Hall and the buried horrors of the children that had lived there and, fearing another attack, he took them from her quickly to pay for the lot.

'In case they don't fit,' he said, handing her the receipt.

Keen to avoid tilting back into a full anxiety attack, he marched straight towards the food hall now, knowing full well that as adrenaline left, hunger would follow. He hit the sandwich fridge and had just grabbed a pastrami and mustard when someone shouted: 'Cam!'

He span, and, on sight, his heart both leapt and sank. He didn't want to see anyone, but particularly not the only person who'd stirred a feeling stronger than politeness from him in years.

In a Roys uniform, holding a crate of bananas, was Jess Tabernacle, her pink hair and silver piercings as eye-catching as her smile.

'You look like shit, mate,' she said, her grin wide. 'You look like a surf pervert.'

He looked down at his dryrobe, suddenly aware of the filth he radiated and the smell that probably came with it. 'Hello. You working?' he asked.

'No,' she said, shifting the crate higher up her hip to roll the banana bunches into the display. 'I just come because I flipping love fruit.' She looked at him with mischief.

Cam flushed at his own awkwardness. 'Fair point.'

She pointed from his toes to the top of his head. 'You in the middle of a busy day?'

'Busy couple of days.' The chemistry was awkward, but real. He felt it crackling like burning paper – but nothing was coming near the overwhelming feeling of pressurised panic. He needed to get away. If he was going to see her again, he didn't want her to see him like this. He needed to reset. Badly.

Jess started arranging the bananas in the display tray, flipping them over so that the widest part of the fingers was facing the customer. 'What are you doing out this way?' she asked, her eyes on the task in front of her. 'I thought you lived out in Neatishead?' Her hair bounced as she chatted, and Cam fought himself not to look at it.

'I needed some bits and pieces,' he replied.

'Do they not have shops in Neatishead?'

'I was passing through, thought I'd stop in here.'

'Ah, so you thought you'd visit the bright lights of Wroxham.'

'No, I…' Cam was feeling the ringing in his head again. He needed rest and solitude urgently, not Jess Tabernacle and that mischievous smile of hers. Worse still, he felt like a schoolkid, floundering with sudden feelings he couldn't explain.

'Just grabbing a sandwich,' he said before walking past her at a clip. 'Sorry, got to run.'

He knew where he was running to now and it wasn't just the checkouts. He didn't even stop to see poor Jess's reaction to his rudeness. Cam was going straight to the pharmacy. He needed his meds and he needed them now.

30

Cam walked into the lobby of Hotel Wroxham looking like he'd fallen off a boat. The man behind the desk stared at him with such uncertainty, it was as if he could see a cloud of green filth following the diver into the building.

Anxiety was punching through him with such bruising speed, he almost didn't know what to say. His mind clawed at handholds, anything he could grasp in the cerebral recesses to give him confidence.

'I have a reservation,' he pushed out, channelling as much of Roger Moore's Bond as he could. Some said those movies were cheesy, but Cam had always felt that if he could just bottle 10 per cent of Moore's suavity in the face of trouble, he'd get through. 'But I'm a little early. Any chance the room is available?'

The man gave him the full top-to-bottom once-over, his eyes lingering on Cam's dirty shoes and the happy dog bustling excitedly between them.

'Busy day at work,' Cam said. 'The name is Killick.'

The man peeled his eyes away to look at the screen while Cam took in the lobby. Soft shades of blue were the main theme, while the perfume of fresh linen sat in the air like a floating blanket. The occasional clink of cutlery came from the double doors behind him, where he knew the restaurant and bar area lay. He began to feel soothed by the familiarity of the place and as the anxiety began to wane, tiredness moved forward to take its place.

'I've got you here,' the man said, looking for a pen to go with the registration form he had in his other hand. 'You're in luck. The room is ready. A junior suite over-looking the river. Dog-friendly of course.'

Cam wouldn't go so far as to say the man was now being friendly, but it was a definite upgrade on the earlier vibe. After the key and registration forms had been swapped and signed, Cam walked into the bar and asked for a straw. The barmaid gave him one with a look of amusement, and he went up to the second floor, following the signs for his room number.

As soon as the door was open, Nala jumped on the double bed.

'Don't you pee on that,' Cam said to the dog as he struggled through the door with his hands full. Instead, Nala curled up just below the fluffed pillows.

Cam sat at the foot of the bed, devoured his sandwich and took in the surroundings. The room was clean and spacious, while beyond the sliding glass door and balcony, the river rolled by, bejewelled by swans.

His head, his heart, his very blood were clearing.

But it had scared him. Being on the cusp of blacking out in that clothing store reminded him just how fragile his well-being was.

After the sandwich, Cam decided begrudgingly it was time to top up his medication once again. Going cold turkey had worked out surprisingly well, but he'd been on the go that whole time, his mind always occupied, his hands always full. And when the adrenaline had faded, the bad had come back, heavy and hard. Now he had to face something he'd come to struggle with.

Sleep.

Knees together, he carefully unpackaged the medicines, popping them onto the bedspread so he could make a clear count. Everything prepped and accounted for, he put them all in his mouth before he could talk himself out of it. He swallowed without the need for water and started on the second sandwich to force the pills down.

Hunger solved, Cam walked into the bathroom, stripped and ran the shower. After giving Nala a thorough rinse, he got in himself, and stayed there for fifteen full minutes as the water punched the chill from his body and he scrubbed all remnants of dirt away. The one thing he couldn't get rid of, however, was the funny taste in his mouth he'd picked up in the lake by Brindley Hall. Water like that, so thick and dirty, tasted like an ancient coin found in a sewer drain. The taste would be there for days.

After the shower he ran a tepid bath without adding any soap or bubbles. Picking up the drinking straw he got from the bar, Cam lay down in the water.

'Let's have a sleep now,' he said. Nala was unable to find a spot like the one she liked at Haven Cottage, so she lay on the floor, huddled on the bath mat next to the tub. Cam stroked her, then rolled back, sinking beneath the surface of the water, and felt the glorious pull of submerged sleep come for him in a matter of seconds.

October 1987

I can't remember ever being this excited before. Tonight, me and Tommy are going out with Mum and Dad to one of the special parties. I'm so excited that my fingers are tingling and my ears are itching. We've been driving for twenty minutes now, and Mum says we're nearly there.

The lights on the road whizz by in the darkness. We are in the back of Dad's Jaguar, which I think is his favourite car. He keeps standing on the front porch to look at it on the drive.

Father's car is a jaguar, and pa drives rather fast.

We are going to the mayor's house. I'm going to tell the mayor's wife all about my horses at home, and about how I'm going to be a famous jockey at Newmarket one day. I'm going to tell her now that she should remember my name for when I win the Grand National. I'll see if she can help me name the horse that's going to win.

I can't stop smiling, so much my cheeks hurt.

I turn to Tommy. He's staring out the window, watching the street signs go by. He's been quiet since we set off, but I think he's just tired. It is late after all.

'Tommy,' I say, and he looks at me. The orange street lights make him glow like a Quality Street wrapper. 'When I get my first racehorse, what do you think I should call it?'

He smiles at me, his grin big and toothy, and says: 'How about Funny Little Girl?'

I giggle. He always makes me laugh so hard I end up needing the toilet, but I can't do that now. But I do manage to ask him why.

'Well, then she can be just like her owner, can't she?'

I laugh some more, and he adds: 'Oh, perhaps we should call it Funny Little Laughing Girl.'

I can't stop laughing now. But Tommy carries on, now doing an impression of the commentary of a horse race. 'And it's Wild Stallion coming up the inside, Wild Stallion a furlong out from the finish line, but here, wait a minute, here comes Funny Little Laughing Girl – and she's got a funny little laughing girl on her back!'

He's laughing. I'm laughing. I feel like I might be sick.

Then Dad turns around, and his voice is so serious my giggles catch in my throat. 'Calm down you two. We're nearly there. If there's any trouble from you tonight, well… There better hadn't be, all right?'

Dad's snappy again, but that's so normal now I don't really notice it. He looks nervous. He's looked like this for a few weeks now.

'We promise, Dad,' I say, immediately trying to forget everything Tommy said to make me laugh.

Now when I look out of the window, I see that things have changed. In all the fun, I've missed that we are turning into a long driveway that has a gate. It has lanterns all the way along, and it looks like a fairy world.

As we travel along the enchanted drive, I think about how jealous Dad must be because our drive isn't as long as this and he does get a bit funny about things like that. When we come out around the bend an amazing house appears. It is lit up like the front of an Advent calendar.

Dad parks next to a man in a funny hat, who walks around to the driver's side. Dad leaves the engine running then turns around to look at us.

'Best behaviour everyone, please,' he says. It looks like he's begging. And as he turns back around, he looks at Mum. 'All the best, darling,' he says to her, in a way that is almost angry. I can't see Mum's face. She doesn't say anything back.

With no more words, they jump out of the front. The men in funny hats open our doors too, and when the cold air comes in, music and lovely kitchen smells comes with it. Something meaty, with gravy.

In my head, there is no way this day could ever get any better. Just me, my brother, my Mum and Dad and this magic evening.

I just wish Mum and Dad felt that way too.

31

Cam woke violently and threw himself out of the water, suddenly on the highest of alerts.

There was noise everywhere.

In his sudden extraction from sleep, he lost all sense of what was happening.

There was a dog barking. A thumping all around him. There was a voice calling his name, but it sounded distant and far away, lost in the thudding of what sounded like helicopter rotors. But he was indoors, naked, on his hands and knees on a bathroom floor, somewhere unfamiliar.

Had he been captured? Had the past finally come back? Or had he never left?

That dog was barking again, and then he saw Nala. He knew her name. He knew that she was his dog. His head hurt from his sudden collision with consciousness and he felt like he was swimming.

Thump thump thump.

And then a voice: 'Cam! *Cam!*'

He ran out of the bathroom into a nice hotel room, wondering where his clothes were and why he had a straw in his mouth.

Why the hell had he been in the bath?

Where was he?

'Are you all right, Cam?'

And then the door was barged open. A woman with pink hair tumbled in, slipping as the door jamb gave way. When she steadied herself and saw him, she turned away with wide eyes. 'Oh my days.'

Cam was suddenly very aware of his nudity.

'Cover yourself up, for crying out loud,' said the woman, darting into the bathroom as Nala ran around her feet in a fit of apparent excitement. Cam didn't know what he was supposed to do. Simply breathing was something his body needed to be reminded how to do. The woman returned from the bathroom with a large white towel and held it out in front of her, covering his modesty. He covered himself and lowered himself to sit on the edge of the bed.

Still, he didn't know who or why she was here.

'Look, I'm sorry about your door,' she said, flustered. 'I was just worried that's all, you weren't replying. I heard Nala barking, and then I heard the splashing.' She knew his dog. It was like he was supposed to know her.

The woman's eyes changed suddenly, widening in shock. 'Oh shit, you didn't try to do something stupid, did you?'

Her hand came up to cover her mouth, and he followed her gaze to the blister packs at the end of the bed. A jigsaw piece fell from on high and threatened to slot neatly into the right place in his head.

'They're normal,' he said, realising as he did so how ridiculous that sounded. He pulled the towel tighter around his midriff. 'I mean, they're normal for me. That's what I usually take.'

He remembered now. His name was Cam Killick, the words bursting through the fog. His memories came back in a sudden rush of cohesion. 'Thanks for looking out for me,' he said. 'I'll pay for the door, don't worry about it.'

She looked at him uncertainly and folded her hands. His cheeks flushed.

Jess Tabernacle had just seen him naked. 'I'm sorry about that, and I'm sorry about… this.' He looked down to his now-covered nether regions.

'Give a girl a heart attack, why don't you,' she replied. Then she lowered to her haunches in front of him. 'Are you all right, Cam? Is everything OK?'

'I'm honestly not sure.'

'What happened?' Her concern was genuine. He looked at her, scouring for judgement, but she gave none. There was only care.

Cam looked away from her, unsure what to say, although now he was coming back together, he knew exactly what had happened. All that medication after days without, then going straight to sleep – underwater of all places – would always be a recipe for serious confusion.

'I dozed off that's all,' he said, eyes on the carpet.

She arched her eyebrows. 'You fell asleep in the bath?'

'Sometimes it's the only way I can sleep'.

They were quiet for a moment. He was struck by the emotion in her face – that she had come looking for him to check he was OK. Then he realised his being here at Hotel Wroxham was supposed to be a secret. He deliberately came here so that no one could find him – yet here Jess Tabernacle was, literally knocking his door down. 'Forgive me, but what are you doing here?'

'Ah, you see, I knew you were a proper weirdo. So when you left the shop, I followed you – to make sure you were all right, of course. You left in such a hurry and … I don't know, you always look so … haunted.' She said this without a hint of embarrassment, like keeping an eye on his welfare was the most natural thing in the world. 'When I saw you coming here, I went back and finished my shift. And when I was done I came to … I don't know, check on you. You're like a wounded animal, wandering about on half-speed.'

Bullseye. Cam bristled at her words.

'I know Darwin on the desk downstairs. He's always bloody there, he never stops,' Jess continued, 'so I asked him which room you're in. Then I heard you splashing about in the bath like you were drowning, so I had to, you know, force the issue.'

'I see,' Cam replied. He suddenly felt so bare, so naked, in both the physical and emotional senses, he wanted the bed to swallow him up.

But then something changed in Jess's eyes. The care was replaced by something else, wild and rising. The change was so quick, his disorientation still so strong that he almost didn't recognise it. It was abject fear — and surprisingly, it brought out of him a sudden urge to protect her. 'What's the matter?'

She said nothing, her eyes wide and staring.

'Jess, what is it?' he asked.

Jess Tabernacle turned and ran out of the room, her footsteps echoing along the corridor.

32

Still bemused by Jess's exit, Cam headed out to the car park, and his van. He felt so embarrassed – sure he had done something or said something so disgraceful she couldn't bear to look at him anymore. However, more than anything, he felt concern. Those titanic shifts in behaviour and mood carried all the hallmarks of someone dealing with exactly the same kind of thing he was.

He opened the back of the van and reached into the shelves for the huge white tarp he used for sorting finds. It often got mucky, but was cleaned in a pinch with a jet from a hose or shower. It would be perfect for what he needed to do next.

As he walked back into the hotel, he stopped by the front desk to own up to the door and offer to pay for it.

'We're going to have to move you a couple of doors along. You're very lucky it's out of season and we've got another suite available.' The receptionist, Darwin, Cam supposed, looked smug and disdainful as he handed over the new key. If he looked any further down his nose at Cam, he'd have gone cross-eyed.

'And *you're* lucky, I'm not going to make a complaint about you giving my room number out,' Cam said firmly. Darwin's veneer cracked, and just as he began to stammer in humbled embarrassment, Cam strode off to the stairs with Nala's claws clicking merrily on the tile alongside him.

In a whirlwind Cam grabbed his things and moved next door, into a suite that was the mirror image of the one he just left. Once settled, he laid out the white tarp on the floor, and pulled the photographs out of the bag one at a time. They were filthy, some still with water trapped under the glass, and it was messy work.

Taking a fresh hand towel from the bathroom, Cam set it on his knee before carefully removing each frame from the fetid bag. They cracked against each other and jangled with the sound of brittle glass as he lay them in rows on the canvas.

By the time he was done, there were three rows in total. Cam looked at the display of photographs, absorbing the bigger picture they collectively portrayed.

They were all in various degrees of decay, but otherwise painted a picture of Freddie Brindley; a man besotted with the glitz and glamour of the highlife. He was handsome, and had a Golden Age Hollywood look to his hair and brow. He would've been extremely suited to life as a celluloid hero himself, if it weren't for the fact that in each of the photographs he was brushing shoulders with people who the camera favoured more. It was as though there were some unspoken acknowledgement by everyone in the image, and the image creators themselves, that Freddie would be the B-side to a more famous A-side. The problem, however, was that Cam didn't recognise many of the people in the photographs.

They were taken with what was clearly a professional camera, with none of those tell-tale condensed giveaways of 1980s disposable camera images. Despite the damage, bubbling colours and smudged muddy edges, the clarity of the images suggested that they'd been taken by a press photographer.

Cam looked more closely across the eighteen pictures and tried to pick out those that he found carried recognition. There were only three people he thought he knew, none of whom he could remember by name.

He hopped up from his makeshift art installation and made himself a cup of coffee. Nala watched him from the bed where she was dozing, one eye following him as he moved. He tossed a treat onto the bed for her, and she made a languid play for it. As the kettle boiled, he looked at the canvas he'd made, the water simmering and bubbling in tandem with his mind.

What was so important about these photographs?

Why were they so sought after?

He reasoned that it had to be the identities of the people Freddie Brindley was with. He'd studied Freddie himself in each of them, and there wasn't anything which suggested troublesome criminal activity – unless said criminal activity was simply proven by association with the characters Cam had yet to identify.

Cam needed extra eyes on this. But he couldn't heave the photos about in this ungainly state.

Coffee in hand, the steam reaching up like bitter tendrils, he took his place at the foot of the tarp and picked up the nearest picture. Using the towel now replaced on his lap, he began the careful process of removing the pictures from their frames and wiping them dry, or clear of mud. The frames would go into the big bins in the hotel car park. The photographs would be easier to transport once flat and pressed together. Far easier to hide too.

Cam found himself fortunate once again, because when it came to photographs, Freddie Brindley had maintained his characteristic of having expensive tastes. Each one of the prints was top quality and on high grade paper, produced to a professional specification. These weren't the kind of prints you got back after you'd dropped a disposable camera into a pharmacy with a one-hour development promise. These were so well produced that the ink had barely run even where the pane had cracked and suffered water ingress.

With a growing pile of dismantled frames accumulating at his feet, Cam worked carefully and methodically, treating each photograph as a work of art over which he had sole responsibility of restoration.

He laid the stack out on the bed. The whole big picture seemed clearer this time, fragments pulling into focus. Along with the three mystery subjects he recognised, he felt a slight inkling of recognition on a further two.

Cam stood, remembering something he'd read about internet searches when you have an image you want to match, as opposed to words. With sudden urgency, he took the photograph nearest to him and held it under the light.

Yes, he thought. *This would be worth a shot.*

He set it on the surface and took out his phone. Zooming in, he took a headshot of the mystery man in the picture – a white, ample-gutted, silver-haired man who would be in the far reaches of old age today. He had a tan, and laughter lines either side of teeth so stained you could take them out and draw with them.

Now that the picture was on his phone's camera roll, albeit somewhat reduced in clarity, Cam felt that buzz of progress once more. Still standing, he clicked through to Google and typed in 'reverse image search'.

Tapping the search bar, he uploaded the headshot of the mystery man. He couldn't look away from the screen as it found a response.

A number of images came back. A lot of them were men who looked similar, but not quite the subject in question. A bunch of other results, thanks to the mysteries of AI algorithms Cam would never understand, were pictures of things that bore no conceivable relevance to the man at all. One such image he'd been gifted was of a china teapot.

But then, on the third row down, he saw him. And underneath the image was the caption, 'Albion Hewitt'.

Of course! The name struck an instant chord with him, and Cam remembered why he recognised the man. Whenever the name Albion Hewitt was referred to on television news bulletins when Cam had been a child, he'd always popped his head up to have a look. It was such a unique name, it had always piqued his interest, in a 'who on earth would be called that?!' kind of way. And now, decades later, Albion Hewitt was popping his own head into the present.

Cam clicked through the link below the image and was taken to another page. Sure enough, it was an obituary in *The Times*, detailing Albion Hewitt's peaceful passing at the ripe old age of ninety-four, back in 2007. The article continued that he was a much beloved Liberal MP, whose work for his constituents would always be remembered fondly. He was also known as a bit of a cad, or maybe that was an uncharitable inference Cam himself made when he read that Hewitt had been married five times.

Politics.

There it was.

A sudden, firm link between politics and Freddie Brindley. It made him think of the boastful arrogance and slippery confidence of the man in the trees on Hickling Broad, who'd orchestrated the destructive search of Brindley Hall. He'd carried the firm, Teflon air of governance.

Cam went to the dresser by the bed, moved his open dive pouch out of the way from where he'd tossed it, and found the complimentary pen and notepad.

He had a name. He had a face.

And now he had a note.

Cam took the photo of the next person he almost recognised and repeated the process on the vanity dresser. Image uploaded, straight into reverse image search on Google.

The results were practically instantaneous, only giving him a second to marvel at the technological advances before it returned an image of a much younger man, with tightly drawn cheekbones, a glittering smile and immaculate hair. No wonder he'd seemed familiar. It was Charlie Safin, boy-genius footballer, once touted as the next great thing in world football and destined for international greatness… Until injury stole the whole lot from him. His career ended at twenty-four years old and he descended, the article told, into a maelstrom of self-inflicted carnage. Drugs, booze, sex, all in numbers the average human being couldn't begin to contemplate. The cruellest irony, Cam thought as he read the piece, was that the injury which killed off his career would only result in him being three months off the pitch today, such had been the advancements in science and sports therapy.

Either way, for Cam this was more evidence that Freddie Brindley was brushing with high society and celebrity. Whether these people were clients or friends was still unclear.

He repeated the process with the third, fourth and fifth photographs.

Another politician, a newspaper editor and a tennis star.

He looked at the five names he'd written down. Five names he hadn't heard in years but were all in the public eye when he was growing up. All were spoken about in articles as party-going – some even carrying the whiff of scandal. Despite the star wattage, it was a motley crew.

Cam picked up the sixth photo to repeat the process again, but when he locked eyes with the mysterious man in this photograph, it hit Cam like a slap in the face. He *knew* this man: a shape shrouded in shadows in the trees; an angry figure pulling himself up from an overgrown lawn. Younger and preserved in a photographer's flashbulb, his eyes were deep brown with wide pupils that seemed to want to give you the truth. His facial features were just a touch too prominent, as if his nose, brow and mouth had been fed into some image editing software and increased in size by 10 per cent. His face was reddened, the skin irritated and sore.

Without doubt, this was the man who had been pursuing him.

Cam repeated his reverse image search procedure and was hit by yet another name he recognised.

Lord Chalmers, Cam thought, the pennies dropping in his head so heavily he could almost hear them. That was why he wanted to keep everything so secretive. Cam's grasp of the national political scene was reluctant, and so far, it had stood him in poor stead – because if he'd been paying attention, he'd have known this man in an instant. Lord Chalmers was once an MP for East Anglia, long serving, multiple re-elections. Even Cam, in his ignorance, knew that. Chalmers was still on the periphery of politics, Cam seemed to remember, now a member of the House of Lords.

He was stunned. That was as high up the political ladder you could climb, save for the top job at Number Ten. No wonder the man had oozed the composure and smooth talk of government.

But what could Lord Chalmers want with some old photographs of Freddie Bindley?

Cam added the name to the list and had to park his excitement at the development as he tried to stick to the task at hand.

The next thing he had to do was establish what further link there might be between the people in the photographs and Freddie Brindley — if there was any dark, secretive business between them. His thoughts then leapt to that old computer in the storage well of his van. What answers might be encased within it? But to extract them, he needed access to a level of tech support he simply couldn't source alone.

Cam drank his coffee and went out onto the balcony, his mind rotating on the facts and whirring to establish the best course of action. He stared at the water that eked by in a fat column of black, dappled by the flickering reflections of the houses on the other side of the bank. It was freezing, but Cam found it bracing.

The best chance at meaningful justice here, whatever that meant, was always going to be with the weight and rubber stamp of the police — even if, at this point in time, they wanted nothing to do with the matter. This story, these new strands… even in its bare threads, was compelling. And it was growing so fast, he felt compelled to share it.

The police would have to take this seriously. And that meant DS Rogers. He needed her intel on this *now* – officially or unofficially.

He went back into the hotel room, picked up his mobile and dialled.

33

It had gone ten o'clock at night when Rogers arrived in the lobby of Hotel Wroxham. Darwin – it seemed Jess was right; when did that guy go home? – gave a surprised glance as Cam ushered her straight to the stairs, fully aware of how, in his short stay at the hotel, he was coming across as a strange and unpredictable guest. Also aware of how nosy Darwin could be, instead of greeting Rogers properly he simply said: 'Let's go straight up, talk up there.' It would've done nothing, he imagined, to dent Darwin's interest, but that was on him for being such a nosy fucker.

As soon as they were in the hotel suite, Rogers huffed moodily.

'Christ, I really shouldn't be here,' she said, hands on hips. She was in jeans and a black jacket, her long blonde hair in a thick plait over her left shoulder. She looked deeply exhausted. Cam hoped that the reason for her demeanour was her frustration at having a dynamite case in play, but a 'don't touch' warning from her superiors. Yet, like any consummate investigator, once the carrot of a lead had been dangled, she'd been unable to resist coming out in person.

'I know, I know,' Cam said, stepping towards the bed. 'But I think I've got something concrete here that I need your help with. Do you want a coffee?'

Rogers ignored his question. She was looking at the photographs all over the bed, Nala lying at the head of them like the proud artist who had put the display together. Cam took a step back and allowed her to take the central position at the foot of the bed.

'What do you see here?' he asked.

With a tone that betrayed the turning of internal cogs, Rogers replied. 'I see Freddie Brindley, with loads of people who were famous aeons ago.'

'Have you ever seen these pictures before?'

'These would all be fresh news to the investigation – if the powers that be hadn't oh-so-intelligently killed the investigation.'

Cam went to the side of the bed and pulled his dive pouch from the drawer. He proceeded to talk her through the events of the last couple of days.

About the group that assaulted him at Haven Cottage.

About what he found on the dive at Hickling Broad, at which point he pulled out the teddy.

About the man who had hidden in the trees and told him in no uncertain terms to leave it all alone.

He went on to talk about his trip to Brindley Hall, and how a group of thugs had come and ransacked the place while he had hidden in the dollhouse.

How they'd been looking for photographs – a pile of which he went on to find submerged in a bin bag in the lake next to Brindley Hall itself.

What he didn't share however, was Jess Tabernacle's visit. It wasn't relevant, nor was he ready to think about all of that just yet – *oh my god, she saw me naked, oh Christ* – let alone talk about it with someone else.

Rogers was quiet and still, except for her eyes as they drifted across the photographs on the bed, the diver's pouch in Cam's hand, the pile of smashed frames on the floor.

After a while, she turned to him. The whole facade of disinterest had faded. 'You never heard me say this, Cam Killick,' she said, 'but you've done an incredible job here.'

Cam felt suddenly bashful, but vindicated. 'Thank you,' he replied. 'But it means nothing if we don't get to the truth – for whoever had this when they were a kid.' He held up the toy dog he'd retrieved from the dive last night. It looked more tired and faded than ever in the dim light.

'This is all stuff the police could have done themselves, Rogers. They should have swept the rest of Hickling Broad for more evidence as soon as the car had come out. The question is why they didn't.'

Rogers reached out and took the teddy. She held it in a careful hand, as if it might explode into dust any second. 'My god,' she whispered.

'The question is, where the hell have they been all this time? I mean, they're surely dead, aren't they? And all *this* suggests' – Cam pointed at the bruising on his face – 'they had to have been killed to keep something secret.'

'Things certainly seem to point that way.'

'Unless they're out there somewhere. Were there ever any sightings after that night? Anybody ever called in with a tip-off?'

'Never...' Rogers looked at him directly. 'Or at least none that ever made the file.' She cocked her head with raised eyebrows. 'I can look into it again, because of course, we now know the file was manipulated.'

Cam nodded slowly, getting the hint, and took the teddy back. 'The question is why.'

Rogers sighed, seeming to weigh up what might come out of her mouth next. 'My hands are tied in a lot of ways. You might see me and think "ah senior cop, must have lots of sway", but it isn't like that. Not at all. The nick's run by paper-pushing box-tickers and yes-men. But... I joined the police with ideas of my own, you know. That I might be able to do something about what happened here. I think that's why I took pity on you,' she said with an apologetic smile. 'It's why I gave you the CID number. Maybe I secretly wondered whether you could do what I couldn't.'

Rogers moved across to the kettle and started making the coffee she'd refused moments ago. Cam, however, was puzzled.

'What do you mean?' he asked.

She busied her hands with the mundanity of the task, but the look on her face was miles and miles away.

'Tommy Brindley was a scout in one of the North East Norfolk districts. I was a venture scout at the time, which is what girls who wanted to join scouts were, before it all became mixed in the early nineties. Us girls were older and helped out. I knew Tommy. Did all sorts with his group – days away, camping trips, the lot.'

Cam was shocked, but somehow not surprised. Rogers continued as she filled the kettle in the bathroom, her voice carrying a momentary echo from the tiles. 'He was such a quiet, sweet kid. But really solid too. He knew his own mind, had a moral compass like you wouldn't believe. I was already umming and ahhing about joining the police by then, but that ... that was the tipping point. The idea that this kid and his family could just beam off the face of the planet. I couldn't get it out of my head. Not that any kid deserves to go missing, far from it, but how could this have happened to such a *good* kid? So, into the police I went.'

She rinsed a couple of mugs while the kettle boiled. 'Obviously when I got there, worked my way into CID, I wanted to look into the Brindley case more than anything else. But every time I tried, I was warned off. The files were kept secret, for the eyes of top brass only. I always wondered why, but never found myself in a position to ask too fiercely.'

'So the Brindley case has always been hands-off?' Cam asked.

'For as long as I can remember.' She poured a couple of mugs of coffee and handed one to Cam. 'Until you, Cam Killick, came along and gave me something to be a lot more bullish about.'

Cam understood what she was saying – the case was personal to them both now – and it brought a determined pride out of him, strong and surprising as a bolt from some lost blue.

There was a knock on the door. Rogers looked at Cam, who nodded.

'You can open it,' he said.

Rogers undid the latch and in walked Gupta and Ferris, the former with respectful awe, the latter with rhino-like bluster.

'We need this scene secured,' said Ferris with overblown authority, before looking at Rogers. 'And who is this?'

Rogers didn't answer, simply turned to Cam with an expression of incomprehension, as if silently asking *and just who are they?*

'Detective Sergeant Claire Rogers,' Cam said. 'Please meet Gupta and Ferris, the hosts of the *Norfolk Unexplained* podcast. I called them when I called you. They've been helping me too – they're also journalists at the *Gazette*.'

'Journalists!' Rogers said, nearly spilling the coffee all over the photographs, before she paused, and eyed them closely. 'It's you two!' She pointed at Cam. 'From the interview that got this berk all hot and bothered. Cam, what the hell are you doing? These two are nutjobs.'

'We're doing what you lot are too scared to do!' spat Ferris.

'Woah, woah,' said Cam, immediately regretting inviting them all here. 'I thought you all knew each other, with the interview and all that.'

'It was on the phone!' Rogers said.

'DS Rogers, I know that your hands are tied,' said Gupta, stepping forward placatingly. 'But we have resources that could help. And we have, haven't we, Cam?'

'That's right,' said Cam. 'They told me that the Belvedere Estate owns a bunch of places, but here in Norfolk, it's just that specific patch of Hickling, and the Brindleys' old home. Which is where I found all this – in the lake by the house.'

Rogers looked across them all in turn.

'We're legit,' Ferris said proudly.

'Clearly,' Rogers said sarcastically. She looked at Cam, then sighed.

She then slid into business mode and surveyed the spread of photographs again. When she next spoke, there was new authority in her voice. 'Collect all these up, we need to get them scanned in. I think we'll have to take this very quietly and run with it ourselves until we've got something completely ironclad.'

'Let's have a look at them first,' Gupta said, as she and Ferris stepped forward. Gupta took her time, while Ferris got on her hands and knees and surveyed them up close.

'One or two of these have got a haloing at the edges,' Ferris said. 'A clear sign of alien contact.'

Rogers looked at Cam as if to say: *really?*

Cam answered quickly. 'They've been under water for nearly forty years. On some the ink has run in the corners. No aliens.'

'So you say,' Ferris replied with her nose still pressed close to the photos.

Cam moved swiftly on. 'This one here.' He pointed at the photo featuring the man who'd been following him the last couple of days. 'Lord Chalmers. We need to know everything we can about him, principally why he needs things to stay secret almost forty years on. Gupta and Ferris, can you do that?'

'On it,' said Gupta, as she leant to investigate the photographs. Ferris, meanwhile, started taking photographs of the photographs with her phone. It took Cam a moment to realise she was scanning them, making digital replicas. Gupta, on the other hand, was speaking into her own phone, holding it out in front of her.

'Killick's hotel room was well-kept but carried the obvious accoutrements of the lone male. Washbag, clothes on the back of a chair, you get the old, oft-drawn picture.'

'What the hell is she doing?' Rogers whispered to Cam.

Before Cam could reply, Gupta looked at them both, and continued speaking into the phone. 'Our presence in the room was met by a lukewarm response from DS

Rogers, something that soon thawed with a little encouragement.' She gave Rogers a cheery thumbs up.

'It's for the podcast. I promised them they could do an episode with official inside info if they helped. It seems they are recording it as they go.'

Rogers looked at Cam in disbelief.

'Don't worry,' Cam said. 'It'll only come out after we – you – close this thing officially.'

Behind him, Gupta carried on speaking. 'DS Rogers quickly began to see how much help and class we brought to the investigation, and we soon got down to work.'

Rogers' glare went volcanic.

'Can we cut that?' Cam asked.

'We didn't agree on editorial,' Gupta said, before mercifully moving back to the photographs. Cam ushered Rogers to one side.

'Think about it,' he said. 'They'll definitely get the real story out, if the police bigwigs won't.'

Rogers looked at him. The fire wilted and she sighed. She was in.

Cam pointed to the pictures. 'Maybe when you get IDs on this lot, you could run it by that guest list you've got for that party at the mayor's house.'

Rogers cocked her brow at him. 'You think I haven't thought of that?'

Cam looked down, embarrassed, but Rogers smiled. 'Don't fret, Cam, I know enthusiasm when I see it. Besides, I already know he's on it.' She pointed at one of the pictures – it was the same picture of Lord Chalmers that Cam had pointed out mere moments before.

Cam leaned over to look. 'Seriously?'

'Yes. Lord Chalmers has always liked a good knees-up, it seems.'

Proof, at last. Chalmers and the Brindley family could be placed together the night they disappeared. Cam could have punched the air. 'Pay close attention to him. The man at Hickling Broad and at Brindley Hall this morning? I'm sure it was him.'

Rogers turned to face him so quickly her plait jumped across to the opposite shoulder. 'Jesus Christ.'

'Yeah,' was all Cam could say, with a weak smile.

'Maybe that's why we've all been told to back off, and it's case closed. If he's involved, a member of the House of Lords, this could have conspiracy vibes all over it.'

Cam nodded slowly, then remembered something. 'The computer in the van,' he said. 'Do you know someone that might be able to have a go at cracking it?'

'If it's as old as you say it is, I think the tech boys will be queueing up to have some fun with it. For them, it'll be like playing with a vintage Mustang.'

'Great.' He paused and put the toy dog back in the pouch. That, he wanted to keep close by. 'Thank you.'

'Look, I'm not far from that pensionable age, despite the youthful exuberance, so save the fanfare.' She smiled and at last looked at him. 'I've worked too hard and for too long to watch my retirement go up in smoke. But…' She glanced almost wistfully at the bed where the photographs had been. 'There's the easy thing, and there's the right thing. What good is retirement when it's full of guilt?'

Cam understood her position and admired her for it. No wonder she had needed a glass of wine to break the news that the case was being dropped. 'I'm assuming that chief of yours will not be pleased if he finds out you're still looking into this?' he asked.

'It'll most likely be my career,' she said. 'But if we find out what happened to those kids, I might be able to live with that.'

Cam nodded resolutely. Excitedly, he collected all the photographs and handed them to Rogers. He'd taken pictures on his phone so he had his own set too, albeit in lower quality.

'I can't wait for our exclusive on this,' Gupta said.

'It's got Pulitzer written all over it,' said Ferris.

'And think of the podcast merch sales,' said Gupta in wonder.

'You two,' Rogers said in school-teacherly fashion. Both Gupta and Ferris stood. 'Don't bugger this up. Don't report anything. You can go mad and sell the rights to Netflix at the end. But until then, everything goes through Cam. Or me.'

'Do you want to be in our WhatsApp group?' asked Ferris. 'I can send you an invite.'

Rogers looked like she was about to burst.

Cam stood to intervene, Nala leaping to the floor, and extended his hand to Rogers. 'Thank you again,' he said.

Rogers cooled and took it. They shook. 'We'll have to handle this carefully,' she said. 'I know a few people that owe me a couple of favours but nevertheless, this has to be more hush-hush than a politician's secret COVID party.'

Cam smiled. 'I'll follow your lead.'

October 1987

This is the fanciest restaurant I've ever been to. It's so fancy that there are three forks on one side of the plate, three knives on the other, and they are all so shiny I can see myself in them. I pick up the teaspoon, but because it's bendy, it makes my face pop like a bug. I can't help but snort with laughter.

'Don't,' says Tommy, next to me. I look at him in surprise. He sounds so serious, so unlike him.

He jabs his head across the table, and I follow where his gaze leads: Dad. He's looking at me funny. Like his face has no expression at all.

Carefully, I put the spoon back where I found it.

Mum speaks, and her voice sounds bright and perky.

'What would you like to eat?' she asks.

'What are the options?' I say. I like that word, *options*. It sounds like grown-up talk.

'Let me have a look.' Mum smiles and takes the menu, which is in a thin red book. As she flicks through the pages, I risk a look at Dad, but he's just gazing out across the restaurant at the door. Is someone else coming? By the look on his face, they wouldn't get a warm welcome.

'It doesn't look like there's a children's menu,' says Mum. 'Excuse me?'

A waiter comes over. He bows at Mum when he arrives, and she laughs nervously. 'What do you have for children?'

'Oh, well, let me see.' The waiter looks at me and Tommy like he's never seen children before. 'Everything on the menu could be done as a smaller plate I suppose?'

'Ah,' Mum says, looking at the menu again. 'You see, I don't think there's anything on there that they would eat.'

'Just order them anything, Maud,' Dad says impatiently, his eyes still on the doors.

'But, *darling*, they won't want it,' she whispers.

Dad looks suddenly furious.

'Well, Maud, sometimes people have to do things they don't *want to*,' and I jump in my seat as he stands up, slamming a big hand down on the table.

'Let's go. Can't even go out for a nice meal without a palaver.' He's flapping about and grabbing our things, and I feel my arm being pulled upwards, out of my chair.

I don't know what happened. I don't know what went wrong. But Mum and Tommy are on their feet too now and Dad is shepherding us all out of the restaurant. As we pass the waiter, I see he looks as confused as I am, hurrying to clear the table behind us.

Dad starts huffing as we get into the street, then he starts to shout — but I don't hear it as I drift away somewhere else, bunching up my fists as I try not to cry.

34

Cam slept better that night.

Yes, he'd still needed to sleep in a full bathtub, this time with a snorkel he'd brought in from the van. But he hadn't woken up with the mad shakes, plucked from a nightmare by burning hands. He simply woke because his mind wouldn't let him rest, hurtling too fiercely between questions, answers and their meanings.

What did Lord Chalmers have to do with the Brindley disappearance?

What links did he have with the thugs who had attacked Cam a couple of nights back?

What was on those pictures, aside from showing simply that Chalmers and Freddie Brindley knew each other, that could cause this much trouble?

The mysteries felt endless, and every supposed answer unlocked only further questions.

For the first time in as long as he could remember, it was Cam who woke Nala, not the other way round.

These were small, cautious steps, and an outlook bolstered by immersion in positive action. Every case of PTSD was different, but whatever he'd been doing seemed to be helping.

It was progress.

It was the kind of progress that made him feel he could do anything. Now in bed watching the early morning through the open window, the river having taken on an entirely different personality in daylight, he reached for his phone and checked through the call register. Found the number that had called him multiple times in a row yesterday, when he'd been asleep in the bath. Jess Tabernacle's number. He called it.

After a couple of moments, it was answered. The voice on the end sounded tired and sleep-croaked, but it was unmistakably Jess.

'Hello?' she said.

'Hi, Jess, it's Cam.'

'Yeah...' she trailed off, before coming back. 'I'm sorry I left in a rush yesterday.'

'I'm sorry I'm calling so early.'

'Oh, it's fine, I'm on my second coffee already, got work in a bit.'

'So ... I wanted to apologise for yesterday. The whole *naked-bathtub-confusion* thing.'

The line went quiet. Then Cam began to hear Jess chuckling, 'Yeah, that was...' she laughed again. 'That was quite something.'

Cam found himself smiling, and a giddy warmth came with it. 'You seemed ... quite upset at the end there. I know it was hardly the most conventional of meetings, but still ... I'm sorry if I did something aside from the whole *naked-bathtub-confusion* thing to upset you.'

She laughed again. 'You didn't. I'm sorry I had to go.'

'It's OK.' He found himself wanting to help. He was so aware of his own frailties, that he felt keenly for others who exhibited similar characteristics. 'Do you want to talk about it?'

'I can't really explain it,' she said. 'Something happened, and it really threw me.'

'What happened, Jess? Do you know?' Cam knew that sometimes, the answers weren't all that obvious, and took some real excavation. But he couldn't think of anything obvious that would have caused it.

'I don't really know. I think. I saw something I think.'

'In the room?' Cam tried his best to picture it, but couldn't think of anything that would elicit that kind of reaction. 'I mean, I wasn't sure about the feng shui either, but still.'

Jess laughed again, and to Cam's surprise, it made him feel positively drunk. 'I think so,' she said. Her voice changed pitch entirely, dropping to reveal unmistakeable confusion. 'For whatever reason, I'm not sure I can talk about it.'

'That's OK.' Cam could feel a heat on his cheeks, but it was not of the usual variety. This one held hope. 'Maybe I could give you a call later, after work?'

'That sounds good.'

Cam was elated. 'Let's do it. But there's no pressure, OK?'

'OK.'

'Oh, one last thing – is Darwin his first name or last name?'

That laugh again. 'I honestly have no idea,' she said. 'That's just what everyone calls him.' Now Jess's voice couldn't hide the fact she was clearly grinning at the other end of the phone line.

'So, he's like Norfolk's answer to Prince, then. Got it.'

'Bye, Cam.'

'Bye, Jess.'

He hung up. And smiled.

By the time he got up and showered properly, he surprised himself again with the thought that he'd like to go downstairs for breakfast. With all the other people who had stayed in the hotel that night. He smiled again to himself – how refreshing not to be poleaxed by negativity all the time.

All right, then: breakfast in the dining room it would be. But it had to be done sensibly. With forethought. Things that hadn't become synonymous with him in recent times. After the adrenaline of finding the car had gone and the heat of action had died down, he'd risked himself in all sorts of ways by going cold turkey on his anxiety medication.

A balance had to be struck.

He took out his usual array of medication and put them on the side of the bed, just as he had done yesterday when he necked the lot. He looked at the tablets, assessing them with the respect they were due this time, and picked them up one at a time, splitting each pill in two. He arranged a half-dose of everything. Let's see how that works, he thought, then jumped up to grab an unused coffee cup and put half of the split tablets in there. The rest, he threw down the hatch.

Again, he felt good about himself. With as close to a spring in his step as he could get, he called Nala to follow him and headed down for breakfast.

Cam found the dining room full of morning sunshine, bouncing off the river outside with glorious abandon. He was wearing a fresh tee and board shorts.

As luck would have it, Darwin was playing maître d' this morning, buzzing about the restaurant with a determined flit. Given that Cam didn't know how long he'd have to stay at the hotel, and knowing that this was the safest he felt in days, he decided to try and mend any bridges he may have left smouldering.

'Morning, Darwin,' he said with a smile and an outstretched hand. With a look of slack-jawed uncertainty, Darwin took it. 'Thanks for your help last night. And once again, I'm sorry about the door.'

'It's quite all right, Mr Killick,' said Darwin, pulling his professional composure back quickly.

'Please, call me Cam,' he replied amiably, and was forced to admit he was channelling a certain seventies James Bond again.

'Would you like a window seat?' asked Darwin. 'The river is looking great this morning.'

'That would be nice, thanks.' Cam was suddenly really enjoying himself. He'd been deprived of such simple niceties for so long, that even this exchange felt like something from a Hallmark movie.

In his subconscious was the idea that what he'd been missing all this time may just have been the drive of occupation, of real duty. So many military men and women came home with an abrupt end to the very thing that made them whole. Filling that hole and finding completion was a trial-and-error process. Maybe for Cam to find his own peace, he simply had to get his teeth into something significant. To feel like he was doing a greater good. It was worth bearing in mind, as he pressed forward on this sudden unlikely road to salvation.

As he was led to his table, weaving between a handful of guests midway through full English breakfasts, he momentarily forgot about the groups of people looking for him. And the fact he had the photographs. *Let them sweat in their ignorance*, he thought. The progress he'd made, combined with the backing of DS Rogers and a sprinkling of the

Norfolk Unexplained podcast duo, had him charged and confident.

He arrived at a table for two, tight to the window, but Darwin took away one set of cutlery without asking. Nala hopped onto the spare chair, span a merry circle and poked her head up to peek over the windowsill. She caught sight of the swans milling about on the water's surface, preening themselves in an apparent nod to their audience.

Cam smiled. Even his dog was happy.

'Tea, coffee, juice?' Darwin placed a menu in Cam's hand as he sat down.

'Coffee with milk, and tomato juice if you have it?' Cam hadn't had a tomato juice in years. He remembered how much he'd loved it and yet, as if a man with his particular mental torment shouldn't be allowed it, he'd starved himself of this tiny pleasure. He'd always done this, a self-imposed penance intimately linked to his own self-worth. *If I'm a waste of time as a person, I shouldn't be allowed nice things.*

Bollocks to that, he thought as he said: 'And a full English,' Cam added with a wink, 'and an extra sausage, if that's OK'.

Darwin sucked in his teeth and took the menu. 'I'm afraid I can't do that one, Cam – but, we do have a special canine full English, provided by a local pet shop.'

'What the hell is in one of those?' Cam asked, bemused.

'I can get you a list?'

Cam put his hand up. 'Don't worry, Darwin, she'd love one, wouldn't you Nala?'

Nala simply looked up at her name, wagged her tail with glee, then went back to gazing at the swans.

The maître d' left Cam and Nala to it, and they both stared out of the window again. The control Cam now felt could signify a new life for him, and a new way forward.

One that could contain happiness and the joy of simple pleasures. Like breakfast in a hotel, with other people, without losing one's mind.

But it didn't take long for everything to rupture. When his coffee arrived, so did another man.

'This seat taken?' his visitor asked, not waiting for a reply before he scooted Nala off like unwanted lint and sat down.

Cam's shield flew up again, his guard immediately ready. He recognised the voice, from both the woods two nights back and at Brindley Hall.

Lord Chalmers had brought the chill in with him. He had a careful mop of brown-grey hair, as if he'd been intermittently staving off the inevitable with the help of a bottle. And now Cam could see him properly, without the hindrance of darkness or distance, he realised how slow he had been not to recognise him sooner.

The man was much older now, almost half a lifetime on from when the picture Cam had seen him in was taken. The sight of him caused a tremor straight up Cam's right leg. Not only had this man been on Cam's tail the last couple of days, but he was one of the men in Freddie Brindley's lost photographs.

'Finished tossing off in the woods?' Cam asked, without humour.

Chalmers grimaced, looking at Cam with controlled hatred. 'We are well past pleasantries,' he said.

Cam looked around at the other people in the restaurant. There were only a handful, and none of them were paying attention.

Chalmers' words were laced with toxicity. 'We've already searched your van. And we're in your room right now. You are so lucky that dog is here and not up there, let me tell you.'

Cam just smiled. He leaned on that imagined Roger Moore confidence like a crutch and thanked his lucky stars that Rogers had taken the original photographs with her. He had to think on his feet as to how to play this, and decided pure misdirection was his best option. 'But you haven't found anything, have you? Because there's nothing to find,' he said. He reached within himself, to find a way to draw this man and his motivations out. 'I knew you'd come knocking eventually.'

This confident approach seemed to unsettle Chalmers, if only fractionally.

Darwin appeared with the tomato juice.

'Here's your juice, Cam. Should I get a place setting for your friend?' He glanced at the visitor and his face bloomed into delighted shock. 'Good grief, it's lovely to have you with us, Lord Chalmers.' The maître d' practically fell over himself to shake hands. 'I'm so sorry, if you'd called ahead, we'd...'

Darwin trailed off, causing Cam to picture Darwin in full morning suit on the tatty red carpet, putting on a uniquely crap champagne reception. Chalmers on the other hand, faced with a bona fide member of the public who wasn't causing him an arse-ache, switched his entire demeanour in an instant, drawing on a career of glad-handing, campaigning, and keeping on as many people's good side as he possibly could.

'Don't be silly, my friend,' Chalmers said with a fifty-grand smile. 'I thought I'd come and surprise my old chum Cam, here. And it's not much of a surprise if you call ahead, now, is it?'

Cam looked at Chalmers with arched eyebrows, and, in a quiet corner of himself, admired the brazenness.

'Quite right, of course,' said Darwin. 'Let me just get you a place setting. And if I may say, it's quite the honour.'

Chalmers put his palms together and bowed his head with nauseous piety. Darwin had barely shuffled away when the politician's face found its previous fire, and when he spoke, his voice had tilted into pure poison. 'As you can see, my power and threats are far from bluffing,' he said. 'And I'm not used to asking for things twice, nor failing to get my own way. You were at Brindley Hall yesterday, we know this.'

The photographs.

What was Chalmers really capable of? He was a Lord, a long-established member of the societal and governmental elite – his influence was surely chasm-deep and wide-reaching. And this situation seemed to scare him.

In turn, that scared Cam too. He thought of the stuffed dog. And Hannah, in the final photo of the family, confused and dragged to the car, her eyes begging the viewer for help. Nobody had saved her.

Cam had to tread carefully, but he found his contempt for Chalmers hard to contain.

'You and your men did a shocking job, didn't you? All that huffing and puffing, only to go away with nothing.' Chalmers' eyes widened, only for a second, before regaining their previous ire. Cam caught the expression in them though – it was underestimation, and it fuelled what Cam said next. 'You see, I was there. I was there the whole time. You were looking for photographs.'

Chalmers offered a mock smile, but the backfoot surprise was still evident.

Cam twisted the knife. 'I've seen them. And I've seen you in them, too.'

Chalmers went volcanic red, his eyes glowing dark in contrast. 'Be very careful what you say next,' he said. If Cam hadn't said something to provoke him, he would be forgiven for thinking that Chalmers was on the cusp of a heart attack. His right hand clenched into a full fist, sitting on the table in front of him like a piece of threatening stone. 'Where are they?'

Cam found that he enjoyed his sudden power over this snake oil salesman – and this too, like so many other feelings of the last few days, carried the tang of recognition. He'd felt this way before, so many times, and had revelled in it then too. That feeling of getting one over on your opposition. He leaned over the table, as if the two men were in the midst of a friendly conspiracy. 'I don't have them.'

Chalmers actually betrayed panic deep in his pupils, and Cam loved it. These weren't the reactions of an innocent party, he was caught in the crossfire of something bigger.

Chalmers leaned forward to meet Cam in the middle of the table and spoke low and hard. 'You are going to tell me where they are, or you're going to get them for me. *Now.* And if you don't, I promise you your life will not be worth living for one more second after this meeting. I will irreparably damage everyone you know – and everyone you've ever met. You have no idea the lengths I will go to. And it's already started.'

Cam leaned back, confident enough to call his bluff. 'It's out of my hands,' he said, then took his coffee. 'And I do not take kindly to being threatened. What you've done in a past life means nothing to me. All I want is justice for the people who got hurt – so we can also play it this way. You get up and leave now, or I make a couple of calls and those photographs get released to the press. They are with someone who has that level of pull as we speak, so don't think I'm bluffing either.' Cam thought about Gupta and Ferris, and just how much joy it would give them if he said they could throw those photos into the public domain like chum into the sea. 'I'm telling you now, it wouldn't take much.'

Chalmers actually smiled.

'You know, I've tried to play nice. I offered you every way out imaginable. Whatever happens next, please remember – I was the good cop, offering you a way to end this peacefully. But you're a fucking idiot. Good luck with what's to come.' Chalmers never broke eye contact with Cam as he pulled a phone out and dialled. 'Do it. He's not co-operating.' And he hung up.

Cam sat in silence, mentally scrambling for a way to tell if this was yet more bluffing. But Chalmers simply held that sickly smile. Cam tried to return it, but his earlier confidence gave way to concern that he might have acted foolishly.

Nobody, he reasoned, got to be a career politician without knowing how deep to push the knife – and when to twist it.

Just as the stare-down became too much, he heard his phone ring in his pocket. He pulled it out to see a number he didn't recognise, although it had the Norfolk area code. He pressed the green button.

'Yes,' he said.

'Am I speaking with Cam Killick?' He didn't recognise the voice on the other end, but it was little more than a rasp.

Cam glanced around the restaurant and outside the window. He couldn't see anyone holding a handset in his vicinity, but he still felt exposed. 'Speaking.'

'I'm bad cop. I'm standing over a friend of yours.'

Cam's blood chilled in an instant. 'Who?' he asked.

'It's a Mr Tabernacle,' the voice said. 'And he's not looking too well.' *Christ*, Cam thought. The old man had been pulled into this, thanks to him.

'Prove it,' Cam said.

A moment passed with the sound of tinny scuffling on the end of the line. 'Hello, Cam,' said a voice.

'Johnjo?'

'Yes.' The tone was full of resignation. As if Tabernacle was embarrassed he was in such a position.

'Have they hurt you, Johnjo?'

All the while, Chalmers smiled with dark smugness.

Johnjo spoke. 'They keep saying they're going to, but I'm not convinced. They're all hot air and very little else, I think. There were more of them than me, that's all.'

A stiff *thump* rang down the phone line. Followed by another. There was a groan. Cam felt sick through every capillary.

'Johnjo?' he said in a panic.

The original voice came back on. 'Do you know what, he's suddenly not so chatty.'

Cam winced. Whatever was happening to Tabernacle, it was his fault.

'What do you want?'

'You need to come here and you need to bring those photographs.'

'Where am I going?'

Chalmers stood, and mouthed, *I'll be off then.* He turned and left, almost colliding with Darwin.

'You're not staying, Lord Chalmers?' Darwin asked, his disappointment all too evident.

'Oh, do fuck off,' said the Lord, still with that rictus at full beam. Cam thought Darwin's face would have made quite the picture – if the voice on the other end of the line wasn't giving him strict instructions and directions.

Cam listened, as he watched Chalmers leave.

He didn't like what he heard one bit.

35

As the dread rose in his gut, Cam began to regret only doing a half-job on his meds. Nevertheless, he charged out of the restaurant, apologising to Darwin en route, with Nala at his heels. That weird dog-friendly breakfast would have to wait, but as always, he had food for her in the van.

He ran up to his room, and found it trashed as promised. Nothing appeared to be missing though, thank god, so he grabbed his dive pouch and dryrobe, and ran back downstairs. As soon as he left the hotel, he could see something had happened to his van. The dread in his stomach tilted sideways.

He ran across the warped asphalt and saw spiderweb cracks all across the windscreen. The passenger window was shattered, and the door was dented, complete with a mucky boot print in the middle of the depression. The rear sliding door was open, and as he reached the vehicle, he could see it had been ransacked. His equipment lay everywhere, strewn about and disorganised. Mercifully, the tyres appeared undamaged, and the vehicle, while banged up, could still be used.

Cam looked around the car park but couldn't see any witnesses. It was out of the way, one of the very reasons he had chosen this place to park in the first place. How had they found him? He looked up and around for security cameras, but in this corner of the hedges at the far end of the car park, saw none. His own carefulness had come back to bite him.

He opened the passenger door, scooped out the glass as quickly as he could. He didn't like leaving the tarmac covered in shards of glass, but wouldn't stick around. Tabernacle needed him.

'In you go, girl,' he said, and Nala obediently hopped up, assessing her seat carefully before she deigned to lower onto it.

Cam didn't offer himself the same level of care, because time really was of the essence. It would take him around an hour to get to where he'd been instructed. He gunned the engine and placed a call hands-free to Rogers – all the while squinting to focus through the spindle cracks of the glass in front of him.

Rogers picked up after a couple of rings and her voice filled the van.

'Cam? If this is about a progress report, you'll have to give me more time, I haven't even had a coffee yet.'

Cam could imagine the detective's sardonic eyeroll and wished he didn't have to go to Norwich and the Constabulary first, since it was in the opposite direction of his destination. The deal was simple. Bring the photographs, and Tabernacle stays alive.

'Rogers, I need the pictures. Things have gone crazy. I've had Chalmers here, my van's been smashed up, and there's some trouble I need to take care of. I can't say much more, because if I do it might jeopardise someone's well-being. I just need to pick up those pictures, and I need to get going.'

Rogers was quiet for a moment, and Cam wondered whether she was angry. But then she said: 'Can I make copies before you get here?'

Cam was relieved. 'That's a great idea. I'm on my way.'

With a stubborn grumble, the van heaved itself onto the road and growled belligerently as Cam hit the accelerator, gunning for Norwich.

36

Cam didn't even see Rogers when he got to the station – he simply asked at the desk for an envelope for Killick. Within moments he was back on the road and heading back the way he'd come, hoping that those he was going to see would understand his detour – and that they hadn't taken out any more of their frustrations on Tabernacle. He hoped, if they got out of the next few hours unscathed, that answers were coming.

Strands of the Brindley mystery were interweaving, but he needed more to complete the tapestry.

As he took Wroxham Bridge for the second time that morning, a thought struck him. What if Chalmers had thought the pictures were in that lost car? When he heard that the car had been found, did he assume that the photos had been found with it? But he still didn't know why the pictures were so valuable – nor why they had been hidden in the Brindley lake in the first place.

As he wound along the A47 towards Great Yarmouth, Cam found himself increasingly on edge, but that was entirely to be expected when you had corrupt politicians and dodgy organised crime figures pulling you this way and that. But considering those complications, Cam was pleased with how his subconscious was reacting. He was still moving forward, working on the fly, adapting to his surroundings and the changing state of play.

The journey to Great Yarmouth took forty minutes from Norwich, and in the mid-morning, traffic was light. Progress was steady, but still not quick enough. Cam jammed the pedal to the floor, the van pushing itself on despite its injuries.

Cam always felt that when driving, you could tell when the coast was getting nearer. The ground began to dip forward, as if the very country was tipping you towards the water – in this case, the North Sea. He knew exactly where he was going because he'd been there a number of times before. Once it had become common knowledge that there was a diver in the area, and especially a diver of Cam's experience, callouts to towns and villages like Great Yarmouth, Cromer, Lowestoft and Sea Palling to retrieve someone or something from the frigid waters that hung around the East Anglian coastlines, were a fairly regular occurrence.

In the case of Great Yarmouth, the summertime littered the old coastal town with revellers in search of the traditional seaside holiday, the clatter of the twopence machines and the steady pour of cold ale. But towns like these had darker sides too, as Cam well knew. He'd had to pull a couple of bodies from the water here. One of them had been wrapped in chicken wire with its feet in concrete. He knew a man who'd been sent to sleep with the fishes when he saw one.

What he hadn't expected was the destination he'd been instructed to reach. It was a tower sixty metres above the arcades and pubs – right on the seafront, overlooking the shore and the distant offshore wind farms. He had never been there socially — hell, he hadn't been anywhere socially in ages before this week — but even he knew that higher up in the tower was a strip club, hailed as one of the country's most unique. Not many pole dancing establishments could boast a sea view.

As he turned right past a dilapidated pub to pass along the dunes, and the sea which he knew was beyond them, he saw a green peak rise just above the rooftops of the pier, maybe a mile and a half further along. Locals called it Snot Mountain, and it was a little green hill that formed part of the pier's rollercoaster. The tower he was headed to was just beyond it.

He glanced to the passenger seat and saw that Nala was now standing with her paws on the window frame, looking out at the beach and its endless sand with a yearning excitement. 'Walkies will have to be later,' he said, as he ruffled her fur.

As he passed Snot Mountain, he turned left after a gleaming American-style diner and parked up next to a small café. Inside, the patrons glanced out of the window with surprised stares, reminding him of the state of his ride. His van possessed zero subtlety now, with its cracked windscreen and dented sides. It looked like it had been picked up by a tornado, thrown around and then unceremoniously dropped with perfect accuracy into a coastal parking space.

Nala looked once at the sea beyond, then turned and saw her master's apologetic expression. Cam didn't need to say a word, and she obediently sloped back through to find her dog bed in the wreckage of the rear compartment of the van. Once again, she snuggled down.

'Good girl,' Cam said. 'Normal service will resume soon, I promise.'

He hopped out, then jogged off down the main street, clutching the envelope like the lifeline it was. He passed the bingo establishments, the knock-off T-shirt stalls, and numerous hollering arcades – all of which begged for the attention of the scant numbers of people that passed – before he arrived at the tower. It stood high over the Landmark pub, which itself was rooted in a half-closed leisure complex. The place was bare: November in a tourist town with no tourists. But the lights still flashed, and the music still played. Seasonal impotence at its best.

He saw the main front door to the building, two panes of glass with handles in them. Above was an unlit neon sign boasting the name 'Sirens', which he had to admit was a good name for a strip club by the sea. It conjured up images of maritime decadence – pirates and sailors alike called to shore into the arms of a certain kind of professional. But any appreciation Cam had for the place was quickly stifled by the sight of two men he recognised through the glass.

His nerves frothed, but Cam held firm and tried to represent as strong and solid an outlook as he could. He reached for the seventies super spy within him and held up the envelope.

The men nodded in unison as the one on the right unlocked the door. Nobody spoke as Cam entered, to join the big, bearded man and Little King Henry with the burnt cheek – two of the men who had battered him senseless the other night at Haven Cottage.

October 1987

I don't know how, but we've been invited to another party. After everything that's been going on recently, and how strange the last one was, I've managed to get myself in a bit of a tizz about it all. I'm so jittery I've got two of the little Pound Puppy babies with me for something to hold onto.

Like the last one, this party is very obviously for grown-ups, but it's still kind of exciting, despite the weird feeling in my tummy. Everything looks so expensive, even more than the things we have in the cupboards I'm not allowed to open at Brindley Hall. There is a television bigger than anything I've ever seen, bigger even than the huge doll-house Dad bought me last week.

I potter around the party, never far from Mum, always with one hand on the hem of her dress. It doesn't take long before I notice that we are the only children here. It's a bit rubbish that they don't even have drinks that me and Tommy are allowed.

I turn around to look at him. He's just behind me, his eyes wide and unsure. It'll be fine, this party. I'm not worried, even if he is. He's got so nervous recently.

Mum follows Dad and another man. He has a face that looks a bit too wrinkly for the rest of him. He didn't say hello to us.

We arrive at a table in a huge posh dining room. If this room was at our house, we'd never be allowed to go in it. On the table there's a huge buffet which looks like it's already been picked through. Bowls of rice with peas and sweetcorn and carrot all chopped up and mixed in, carrot sticks next to bowls of what could be salad cream, and slices of ham rolled up with some kind of spready cheese inside.

'Go on you two,' says Mum. 'Get a plate and fill up.'

We do as we are told, but there's not many things I like. I take a few things anyway because Dad told me not to be rude before we got here. Speaking of Dad, where has he got to? He's wandered off somewhere, I think. With that man I bet.

I know from that last party that Dad's very popular, that everyone wants to chat with him and have their pictures taken with him. I know that Dad works with money and numbers, and Tommy had once told me that Dad looks after money for important people.

Mum scoots us to a seat in the corner of the dining room, and we sit either side of her. She hasn't got a plate for herself. Across from each other, Tommy and I swap glances.

While I crunch carrots, I look at the other people in the room. Some wear penguin suits like James Bond, only they're older than the man in the films. Some wear jeans and flashy leather jackets, their hair sticking out. Some look ill and tired, just like Tommy.

My heart lifts when I see Dad walking over to us. He has that nervous look on his face again and I'm beginning to think he shouldn't keep coming to these parties if it makes him so stressed. He looks at us with a sad face, like he wishes we could go home but we can't. Then he looks at Mum.

'OK, they're still going through with it,' he says. He looks sad and desperate. I don't know what the matter with him is, but I don't like it.

'Even with…?' says Mum, but Dad interrupts her.

'Yes,' he says. 'Apparently, it changes nothing.'

Mum blows out a deep breath and stands up. She smooths the front of her dress and swaps places with Dad. Giving me and Tommy a quick smile, she then walks back through the dining room and takes the first step on the grand staircase.

A man is standing there waiting for her. He looks like a stick insect, a big, long one stood on two legs. He offers his hand, and Mum takes it. The wrinkly faced man is two steps higher than that, smiling at her.

Mum disappears up the stairs.

'God, forgive me,' Dad whispers, standing up suddenly to move towards the bottom of the stairs, but Mum isn't there anymore. I look at Tommy, and his eyes are sadder than ever.

'Is Mum OK?' I ask.

'I don't know. Stay put for a minute.'

Dad is fiddling with something in his jacket, although I can't see what it is – then he goes up the stairs too, very carefully. I look at Tommy again, and he looks back with eyes big as fifty-pence pieces, but he doesn't move.

Neither do I.

We just sit and crunch carrots by ourselves.

But I'm going to stare at those stairs until Mum and Dad come back.

37

'I would love to take your fucking eyes out,' said the bearded bruiser as he and Little King Henry walked Cam deeper into the building. He was, no doubt, the man who two nights ago had cracked Cam across the head with a telescopic bat. 'Jimmy, call the lift.'

Jimmy, the man formerly known as Little King Henry, answered by pressing the button recessed into the wall at the end of the corridor. An elevator door opened to reveal a box-shaped interior clad in red fluff, giving the impression they were about to step inside a fabric whale's heart. There was a mirror embedded in the fluff, in which Cam could see the side of Jimmy's face where Cam had stuffed the flare in. There was no bandage today and the skin was angry, boiled and puckered, with pus weeping down his cheek.

'Doesn't look so bad,' said Cam, but all that did was earn him a gut shot from Jimmy, who reached low like Mike Tyson and swung so hard into Cam's midriff that he was sure his knuckles grazed his spine. Cam buckled, but didn't go down.

Jimmy sighed happily as if a demon had just been purged and said: 'Sorry, Danny, you know he was asking for it.'

Cam coughed and spat on the floor. He looked up at Danny. 'Jimmy and Danny. Bless, you sound like a couple of kids' TV presenters.'

That earned a kidney shot, and Cam felt nausea crash through him in heavy green waves. But deep down in his brain, away from the plight of his body, he was revelling in this. Even though he was getting the shit beaten out of him, he felt some modicum of control – even if only over himself. It was refreshing, new and old all at once, like he'd met back up with the old days at last. He found he loved it.

As the lift lurched heavenward, Cam thought he might throw up for real – but he swallowed bile and stood up straight, wincing and smiling at the three men. 'Nice shot, Danny,' he said.

While the lift ascended, Danny stared a hole into Cam. 'You know you're nothing without those photographs,' he said with a snarl.

But Cam's smile wouldn't be broken. 'That depends how much you think I've told the police.'

For some reason, Cam's threat didn't land. Instead, Danny's grimace turned into a smirk. 'We ain't worried about that,' he said.

With Danny and Jimmy on each shoulder, Cam rode the lift the rest of the way in silence.

When they got to what he guessed was the top, the doors slid apart. It was darker in the corridor than it was in the crimson lift itself. He was ushered roughly out.

At the end of the corridor were black double doors and an empty check-in desk. There wasn't any music playing, and the whole atmosphere was strangely pressed and close, yet somehow, still vacuous. Danny opened the double doors and Cam was shoved through, the envelope still in his hand.

The first thing he was hit with was a vast, floor-to-ceiling view of the sea. It was slightly dimmed, as if being viewed from behind huge sunglasses, and Cam realised the windows were tinted. He supposed he understood why, because just in front of those windows was a stage with three poles on it. And strapped to the centre pole, his legs splayed on the floor, was Tabernacle.

'Hey up, Cam,' he said.

'How are you hanging in there?' Cam replied, as he was pushed into the centre of the room. The room itself was a darkened space with a neon heartbeat, pulsing along in a soft, undulating rainbow. The carpet was an endless interpretation of the deep, dark ocean, with rolling waves frothing in 2D everywhere you looked. A bar squatted over on the left, shutters down on all but one left-hand segment, while on the right was a series of doorways with curtains across them. The main area of the floor was a sea of booths, with a selection of chairs around the base of the stage.

'Oh, you know, surviving,' replied Tabernacle. He didn't look too badly hurt, though his hands were bound to the pole behind his back and Cam thought he could see some purple shading around his jaw.

'Not my usual choice of entertainment,' said a voice to Cam's immediate left. Cam swung to look, and saw that in a booth towards the bar, sat an old man. 'But needs must,' he said with a craggy smirk.

The man wore a long black coat and a blue shirt that, even from here, Cam could see was adorned with a ketchup stain. His face seemed to melt to his chin, sagging cheeks hanging limp down the sides of his face like old egg whites dried in the sun. Cam thought he looked half-dead, his eyes purple marbles looking at him from the possible afterlife. Cam did, however, recognise the voice from the telephone. This was the man who had called and commanded him here. Bad cop.

'I am Tyrone Travis,' the man said. 'Thanks for coming.' With a frail hand, he plucked a small tumbler from the table and sipped clear liquid through a straw.

The setting and circumstances confirmed it, guiding Cam not to be fooled by any of the man's perceived frailties. Cam remembered the good cop, bad cop routine Chalmers had been running early with this man on the phone. This guy was evidently backbone to his threats, and the black heart that would execute them — even murder. But was he involved with what happened to the Brindleys, or merely the politico's hired help?

Cam took the lead and walked towards Travis, but as soon as he left the group behind him, hands on his shoulders slowed him down. 'I suppose I've got you to thank for the beatings I've been taking the last couple of days?'

'That would be right,' Travis said, a trace of venom polluting the words. Cam studied the man, trying to work out if he'd seen him in any of the photographs that had once hung on the walls of Freddie Brindley's office. He couldn't place him. Whether that was because of the number of years that had passed — some of which evidently hadn't been kind to Tyrone Travis — or if he was indeed absent from the photos, he didn't know. But he felt sure that if he had been in those photographs, he would've noticed. Instead, he was left with zero recognition, just guesswork and his own bravado.

'He's a loan shark, Cam,' said Tabernacle hoarsely. 'Or at least he was. Everybody knew him.'

Cam filed that information away and looked back to the old man.

'Who made you the arbitrator of old problems?' Travis asked. He took out a vape pen and checked the cartridge with a shake. He then took a deep pull from the spout and blew thick white smoke high over his head. Cam caught a note of blueberries in the swirl.

'Good story though, isn't it?' Cam said. 'And everyone loves one of them.'

Travis coughed up what had to be a vital organ, then reset himself with another deep drag from the vape. 'It is a story that should never have seen the light of day again.'

'You're not one for resolutions then? Getting justice for kids that were hurt a long time ago?' Cam knew he was prodding the bear here, but couldn't resist getting a dig in. These people had been dogging him for days, with the threats and beatings – but when all the chips were down, they were on the wrong side of a history that needed telling.

'What happened to those bloody people couldn't have happened to a more deserving bunch.' The malevolence dripping from Travis's words was unmistakable.

'Doesn't sound very much like a tragedy when you put it like that, now does it?' Cam replied.

Travis dismissed his jibe with a flick of his head – as if to tell Cam that he had no idea what he was talking about. Then he changed direction completely. 'The pictures in the envelope?'

'Yes,' said Cam, thanking the heavens Rogers had made copies. Danny ripped the envelope from Cam's hand and took it over to Travis.

'Here you go,' Danny said to the man.

The old man took the envelope and very carefully pulled it open. The room was silent apart from the soft tearing of paper. Cam glanced at Tabernacle, who looked back at him hopefully. Cam nodded once.

'What the fuck are these?' said Travis, leafing through the photographs in his hand. His face was bent with disgust.

'They're the photographs you've been after, the ones from Brindley Hall.'

'I don't know what the hell these are, but they are NOT the pictures I'm after. I've never seen these before. Where are the real ones?'

38

Cam stared at Tyrone Travis dumbly. The old man looked at him with pure hatred, and threw the prints across the table, splaying them across the sticky surface.

'This is the moment when you get on your knees and tell me where the real photographs are.' Travis said. 'Because there a lot of places in this town where two bodies can get washed out forever.'

Looking for answers, Cam shot a glance at Tabernacle, but Tabernacle could only look back at him with wide eyes, pleading for a resolution that wouldn't involve a watery grave. Danny and Jimmy took Cam's arms and dragged him to Travis's table. Cam was still too stunned to fight back when his right arm was thrust high up his back, causing him to grit his teeth so hard they could smash. Danny followed behind, before pushing Cam's head down onto the table top, pressing his skull into the cheap plastic of its surface.

'Where the fuck are the real pictures?' hissed Danny in his ear.

Cam's jaw was pressed tight into the tabletop, but he managed to find a handful of words. 'These are the pictures from Brindley Hall, I promise you.'

They were — he'd retrieved them himself. His brain wasn't deceiving him, whatever state it was in. It definitely happened … although … had he been pushed in the wrong direction? Had he been used? Had … *Rogers*?

Travis stared at him, pointing with a finger that kept stopping mere inches from Cam's eye. 'You play games in this business, you get hurt. You have no idea what I've done to people who have done far less to me. And every second you carry on this game is another hour of hurt coming your way. I'm talking about the kind of scarring, the kind of cutting, that makes a man beg on his knees for a bullet to end it all. And if you think it's bad what's coming to you…' Travis slowly lifted the fingers of his left hand and pointed at Tabernacle up on the stage. 'It'll be nothing compared to what I'm going to do to him — and I'm going to make you watch every second of it.'

Cam couldn't see Tabernacle, couldn't even move his head, but he didn't doubt a single word Travis just said. 'What are the other pictures?' he managed to say.

'So, you're going to play on with the charade?' With that, Travis pulled out a long knife from somewhere beneath the table. It was bent at a shallow angle in the middle, like a machete that had been trodden on. 'Army boy, aren't you?' Travis said. Cam didn't answer, but Travis was positively foaming to continue. 'I lent an army boy some money once. Not that much, but enough to get him in trouble. Boozer, gambler, the same old sad story. When he couldn't pay up, I went to see him, and he offered me his most valuable possession as interest on the deal. This blade. A kukri, the favoured weapon of a particular Gurkha who had saved the old boy's life in Brunei. Only he didn't pay up. And I had to reacquaint him with the old thing. And boy, could I see why he liked it. Like hot scissors through plastic.'

Cam, while he wasn't scared for himself, was terrified for Tabernacle – and for Jess. Her father's well-being was hanging in a balance that could all depend on what Cam said next.

'I'm serious,' Cam said. 'These are the only pictures I found at Brindley Hall. They were sunk in the lake … I thought they had to be the secret pictures that you were looking for.'

Travis laughed, and it sounded like a flock of vultures taking off before hitting a window. 'I guess this means you'd have me believe you're in the clear. No threat to me at all – right?' His eyes glowed like purple stones through the white smoke he pumped out with industrial diligence.

Cam was genuinely dumbfounded, and couldn't hide it. 'I mean it. I was wondering why everyone was so excited about them myself.'

Travis seemed to consider this, before smirking humour-lessly. 'Then all I've got to worry about is you two loose ends then, isn't it? All I need to do is quieten you two troublemakers, and this all goes away.' The finality of the threat sat in the room like a lead weight.

The air felt like it could shatter. Cam couldn't stand to let it crack further.

'The police will come looking for me,' he said. 'They know I was coming to see you.' He was abruptly dragged up, and able to breathe deeply for the first time in a few moments. The release in his arm felt like a gift.

He took a few deep breaths as the older man shuffled to the edge of the booth. 'I don't give a frosty shit about the police,' Travis said as he gingerly pulled himself up.

Danny made a move as if to help him, but seemed to think better of it and stopped a stride short. When he was finally out from behind the table, Travis drew himself to full height, and it stunned Cam. He seemed to just keep getting taller. When he'd been hunched in the booth, his stooped back had given off the impression of a man who wouldn't come up to Cam's chin. Now, he stood a good few inches over Cam, bearing down on him – the Grim Reaper in wrinkled human form, complete with curved blade. 'Do you think a man like me got all this without having the police onside?'

'If you mean a sticky-floored strip club in a dead-end seaside town, I don't think it's the flex you think it is.'

The milky film over Travis's glare seemed to evaporate, leaving pure fury in his eyes. With surprising speed, he swung for Cam's stomach. Cam, having already been soft-ened up, wasn't looking forward to how the impact would land, but he was curious despite himself to know how much punch the old man packed.

Turned out that looks had once again had deceived him.

Pain arrowed his liver in half: what the old man lacked in power, he made up for in accuracy. The two men on either side had to hold Cam up to save him from falling forward – then Travis grabbed Cam by the hair and pulled him towards him.

'You don't seem bothered about your personal safety,' Travis said. 'You're only a bit bothered about his.' He pointed at Tabernacle. 'But I know he's got a daughter. Jess, isn't it? I think maybe she could do with an introduction to this knife too.'

Travis leaned forward and bared his teeth to speak again, but Cam's mind had already gone white-hot with rage. He went with the momentum and lunged forward to meet

Travis with as much ferocity as he could muster, aiming a vicious headbutt at the bridge of his nose.

'Dad!' shouted Danny. *Ah,* thought Cam.

The crunch was immediate, the claret spontaneous, geysering this way and that, but Cam didn't rest there. Bruised and on edge had always been his favourite place to be.

Danny moved towards his father, his attention pulled from Cam. The son grabbed the old man to stop him from falling back, and the shock factor of Travis's nose exploding gave him the edge on Jimmy. Cam ripped his hand from the loosened grip and swung it, flat palmed, into Jimmy's throat.

Danny realised what was happening so Cam went once again for the old man, Danny's weak spot. He pushed Travis with all his might back towards the booth. When he hit the table, he rolled over the top, and landed in a folded heap on the bench itself, sending the kukri bouncing off behind the booth and into the recesses of the club with a clank of tumbling steel. Cam almost felt bad for wishing the old fart had bust a hip in the fall. Jimmy was coughing and spluttering, but Danny was free now, and the most dangerous threat.

Danny rugby tackled Cam hard through his already maimed midriff, those tattooed angel wings around his neck flying right through him, and they both crashed into a table and chairs, sending tea lights flying and chunks of plastic cracking off in shards. It hurt more, Cam thought, because they'd gone clear through it. If only the old man hadn't been such a tight arse.

Jimmy was regrouping, murmuring unintelligibly through his mangled throat. Danny pulled himself to his feet though in obvious pain.

'You're a fucking dead m—' he said, but his spitting obscenities were broken by a loud clang. Cam looked up to see Tabernacle holding the entire length of a stripper pole. It appeared to be the one he'd been tied to, and he was swinging it round his head with a red face. He started jabbing it at Jimmy, poking and prodding it like a harpoon. At the end of the pole, swinging back and forth, Cam saw the bolts which had been ripped clean from the ceiling – revealing that either Travis's frugal nature extended to all fixtures and fittings of the establishment, or Tabernacle was possessed with a brute strength as yet untamed by age.

At his feet, Danny lay unconscious, a welt on the side of his head already making real progress, while Jimmy danced frantically back out of the pole's range.

Cam got up and started to circle the last villain standing.

'Do you want a beating?' said Cam, but it came out with much more of a gargle than he hoped. Jimmy didn't look so sure, glancing around at his fallen comrades. As if deciding none of them were conscious enough or lucid enough to judge his cowardice, he put his hands up. 'On the stage,' said Cam. 'And carry that old bastard with you.'

After dragging Travis and Danny up onto the stage, he instructed Jimmy to sit at the far pole. Tabernacle stood over him, holding the dismantled pole over his head, ready to brain him at a moment's notice. Meanwhile, Cam searched for something he could tie them up with, and found it on the underside of the stage itself. Right at its public-facing edge was a long rope of blinking strip lights, soft flashing reds pulsing like he was holding the tentacle of a transparent sea organism. He yanked the LED rope from its fittings and tied all the men together around the far pole, and with their belts bound their hands behind backs. Happy with his work, Cam left the two unconscious men to slump against Jimmy, who was jabbering in his ear.

'You know you're dead, don't you?' he said. 'And everyone you know. They're all *dead*.'

Cam cracked him one with a tired, thick fist, making a trio of slumped bodies up on the stage of Sirens. Tabernacle moved to stand next to him and finally dropped the pole with a metallic clunk. 'We should really call the police,' he said.

'No,' said Cam, standing over the men. 'They keep talking about being in with the police, so it's not gonna make any difference to the legal situation.' He thought about alerting Rogers but decided against it. As much as it pained him to think it, he just didn't know whether it was safe to do so. In any event, he and Tabernacle had handled this. This threat had been temporarily neutralised. Travis surely wasn't going to the police, so neither would he.

'No,' said Cam, 'I think I like the idea of this particular establishment's employees finding them and these tough boys having to explain how they had to get rescued by a bunch of girls in their skimpies.'

Tabernacle grinned. The old man was flushed, but alive, his eyes bright with the thrill of it all. 'I like the sound of that, too.'

As he spoke, Cam marched across to the booth – the one that Travis had been using as a throne. The photos were still there, splayed about like oversized pieces of confetti. Even with a quick glance, he could see they were the same images copied from the one stack he'd recovered from Brindley Hall.

He shuffled through a few just to be sure. He was convinced they were the same. He scooped them up and pocketed them.

So ... just what had Travis been talking about? If these weren't the *real* photographs that had caused so much trouble, what were?

39

Claire Rogers didn't quite know how she'd come to investigate her own chief, but somehow it had happened. She sat in her office, waiting for news from the tech boys down in the basement – who had been utterly thrilled when she walked down there with the old Apple Mac and a challenge. That lot had done her a few favours recently, most notably working overtime to bring down a couple of clowns who'd decided that they were going to use a houseboat to conduct an online insurance scam. They thought, because they were mobile, that there'd be no fixed IP address, and that it would be harder to triangulate their position. They'd guarded it with a ringfence of firewalls and VPNs, whatever they were, and these funky-smelling lads in the station basement had vaporised the lot. When Rogers walked in with the Mac, she thought she was going to have to ask for another favour. But when she saw those eager faces, she quickly recalibrated her approach:

'First one to get into this wins a large fish and chips from next door. Sauce optional. Salt and vinegar also optional, but I'll think you're a dick forever if you say no. And don't even think about asking for gravy.'

The boys had swarmed over the machine, and she'd left them to it.

Which left her to head back up to her office, which she'd taken a serious dislike to since her own force seemed so complicit in brushing the truth into darkened corners.

The copies of the photographs from Brindley Hall lay all over her desk, and she gave them all a detailed search with a square magnifying glass she'd begrudgingly bought to solve sudoku with. She combed over every detail, every shadow, every morsel of information she could glean. It was like prospecting for gold, only indoors and really boring.

But in the corner of one of the pictures, she noticed someone that simply didn't fit.

In a picture of Freddie Brindley arm in arm with a soap star whose name she had zero interest in, she'd noticed a man over Freddie's shoulder. He was in a leather jacket, with a red stripe along the sleeve, his hair spiked and coiffured. The age was much reduced, but the smile told the truth. It was the same one she'd looked at so much these last two days.

It was her own chief, Gary Hilton.

Now, it might be coincidence. It could be a quirk of a fate with a very naughty sense of humour.

But DS Rogers believed in neither of those things. Not when it came to crime. She believed it kept her closure rates high, but kept her safe too.

So, her own chief, the one who'd torpedoed the Brindley matter when more questions needed answering, actually used to hang about with some of the key characters in the case.

No wonder he wanted the case dead.

Fearing that either Rylance or Hilton himself might burst through the door asking how that bloody parking ticket bollocks was going, she collected all the photographs again and arranged them into her copy of the Brindley file. She approached it fastidiously, labelling everything to perfection, not letting anything come to chance when it came to going for a conviction – if the day ever came.

With the whole lot safely locked in the drawer, she opened up her computer and found the chief's bio. She read through it, then pulled up what she knew about Freddie Brindley. She compared schools, sports clubs, accolades and employment. Nothing matched.

Then she tried it with Lord Chalmers.

And three times, their bios matched.

Once at primary school. Then again in the scouts (of course).

Then again at university.

Hilton and Chalmers were old chums.

'Diddling bastards,' she seethed, as she started a new document compiling information on the two. She set the save point to the machine itself, not the station intranet. It went against protocol, but she thought protocol must be used to getting shoved by the wayside around here recently.

Her angry typing was broken with the announcement of a text.

Voila.

Where do you stand on curry sauce?

40

By the time they got back to the van, Cam was needing Tabernacle's help with every step. He now matched
his van in looking like he'd been in a road traffic accident. Ignoring the stares of the onlookers outside the café,
Tabernacle posted Cam into the driver's side, and was
greeted warmly by Nala, who jumped up between the
seats to give the old man a proper welcome.

Cam's head rang like broken church bells, and his ribs
felt like a xylophone thrown down the steeple stairs. It
would probably mean a lot of trouble in the long run,
what they had done, and in terms of personal safety, they'd
probably have been better off taking all three men and
throwing them off the tower to land in the promenade.
But he just wasn't built that way and wasn't prepared to
fully tilt himself at genuine darkness.

As soon as Tabernacle had got Cam in and settled,
he immediately turned back. 'I'm getting us a hot drink,' he
said, nodding at the cafeteria in front of him. 'How do you
take your tea?'

'Now?' Cam asked with exasperated surprise. Getting
away from the vicinity was an absolute priority, but
Tabernacle looked like being denied a warm cuppa was

the greatest affront. 'A builder's tea,' Cam said, relenting, as Nala turned her attention to her owner. She tried to lick at the bruising that was forming round his cheekbones and temples, but he brushed her away. Even her enthusiastic tongue would hurt.

He started the engine while he waited and tried to have a moment simply to himself.

Tried to breathe, tried to recalibrate.

But, given the circumstances, it was damn hard.

Leaving those men alive would surely bring them back for revenge. He could go to the police, but given Cam's suspicions that they were in on keeping the Brindley mystery hush-hush, he'd be damned if he was doing that. He didn't want to be swept under the carpet like everything else. He could speak to Rogers, but she was only one person against the entire police machine. There would be a time for that, Cam was convinced – but it wasn't just yet.

They needed somewhere to lie low, if only for a short period of time. Hotel Wroxham was out, and he guessed Tabernacle's own home was out too. Haven Cottage was a no-go, so that meant checking in somewhere else.

Tabernacle reappeared with two steaming takeout cups and put them in the cupholders. He took a couple of moments to put an inordinate amount of sugar into his own drink, seemingly unaware of the urgency of their predicament. Cam didn't know when Sirens opened, but as soon as it did, those men would be found. And if they were worth any of their promises, even only a fraction of them, then the first thing they would do was go after Cam with the illest of intent. Tabernacle too, and Jess, god forbid – but all parties really knew that Cam was the main antagonist of this particular story.

The older man took his seat next to Cam and reached around to adjust the seat lever. He jutted too far forward, cramping his knees, then pulled it back, his eyes staring on an object on the dash. 'Ah, Jess used to have one of those. I think she still does.'

Cam's heart about stopped. 'What?' he said in a low voice.

'Jess, my daughter. You met her, didn't you? She had one of those.'

Cam couldn't speak. His throat, lungs, everything; nothing had air. He followed Tabernacle's eyeline, to the little stuffed dog poking out of the dive pouch. He'd just been carrying it about as a totem of the little girl he was trying to find. It had been by his bed in the hotel room when Jess broke down. It was in the corner of that room, right where she was looking. It had been on the bedside table.

Oh my god. I found it at Hickling.

The little girl, Hannah Brindley, had been carrying two in that famous final picture. Two dog teddies.

Cam's mind was obliterated. But he had to keep moving. It wouldn't be long before Travis and those thugs were found and freed.

Trying to keep his head in the game, Cam guided them out of the car park and onto the main street of Great Yarmouth. Cam opted to go the exact same route that he'd come in, for fear of getting stuck in the back streets and one-way systems that he wasn't completely familiar with. A clean getaway was crucial, as that tower watched them leave in his rear-view mirror like the bloody eye of Sauron – and all the while, Cam's blood fizzed with the anticipation that finally, answers were emerging at last.

November 1987

The house is strange. There is a funny feeling right through it. I think it might be haunted. That now we've been here for a little while, the ghosts have got comfortable enough to show themselves.

I don't like thinking about it, especially not now I'm in bed. My room is lovely, but it's big. Almost too big for me, in the same way that I feel the house is a bit too big for us all.

Ignore it. Ignore it. I hold Pound Puppy tight and look into those downturned eyes. The lights in the room seem too soft. I have a night light on, but it just makes big shadows everywhere.

I wish Tommy were here. At our old house, we shared a room, and in the night, if I was awake like this, I could always look over at him from my bed. If his eyes were open, he'd smile at me. If they weren't, I could hear him breathing – and that by itself, would be enough to let me know there was nothing to be scared of.

My door handle creaks.

I spin in my bed, my heart smashing a hole in my chest, and watch the round brass knob twist. I'm going to be sick; I can feel it – when Mum walks in. My arm is reaching for her before I even know it's doing it.

'Hello, darling Hannah,' she says.

There are tears in my eyes, but they're of happiness and relief instead of anything sad. 'Hi, Mum,' I say.

'Are you struggling to sleep, love?'

'Yes.' My voice cracks.

She opens the door fully, walking fast like she always does where we, her children, are concerned.

'Shall we have a story? What shall we read?' She sits on the edge of the bed, and flicks through some of the picture-books on my bedside table.

'You pick, Mum.'

'How about *Mr. Men*?' She asks, snuggling beneath the covers next to me. I smell her and feel her, and I know I'm OK. She's holding *Mr. Greedy*. 'Oh, look, this one could be about Dad.'

I giggle because I know she's only teasing. 'Why were you awake, Mum?'

Mum doesn't say anything for a moment, before: 'I couldn't sleep either, darling.' Carefully, I look at her. Her eyes are full of tears.

'Are you OK, Mum?'

'Yes, darling.'

'Are you sure?'

'Of course. I'd do anything to keep you safe, you know that don't you, sunshine?'

'I do, Mum.' I squeeze her tight.

'So, let's see what Mr. Greedy has been up to.' She opens the book and starts reading, but I'm not listening. I'm still looking at her eyes. She looks so sad. Like everything in the world is wrong, but she's keeping a brave face on her for me.

But I've seen what's been happening at home. I've seen how everyone has become.

Silly me, I think. This house is haunted after all.

The bad things that keep me awake at night are what is happening to our family.

The ghosts are us.

41

Throughout the rest of the journey, the silence between them was a mass so thick you could touch it. Cam saw a sign for Horning, short of Wroxham by a couple of miles, and took it. If one thing would get Johnjo Tabernacle talking, it was the loosening massage of booze. Horning was a small riverside village dotted with three pubs, a newsagent, a post office and a couple of boutique-style gift shops. It was primarily known to tourists as the place where you could take boat trips along the river Bure on a Mississippi riverboat called the *Southern Comfort*. A pub sign read the Heron's Reach, and Cam parked just along from it, next to a village green packed with honking geese.

'I think it's time we had a chat about Jess,' he said.

'My daughter?' Tabernacle replied, as he looked out of the car window at the pub.

'She came to see me, and it was … interesting,' Cam said.

'When was this?' Tabernacle laughed, turning his body towards Cam now. His surprise was soft, genuine.

'Yesterday, at the hotel in Wroxham. She had a very distinct reaction to that teddy.'

Tabernacle went silent.

'It sent her into a panic attack, it seemed, a really deep psychological event,' Cam continued, his eyes flicking between Tabernacle and the road as he tried to read his face.

The old man avoided his gaze and turned to look out of the window.

'Shit,' he eventually muttered into the glass.

'Shit,' replied Cam.

Tabernacle sighed, but it didn't last. He turned back, a man with his mind apparently made up. 'Well, it would do,' he said. 'Considering it was hers.'

Cam was nothing short of electrified. As revelations went, this was staggering, but to hear it said out loud…

Anything to do with a mystery of missing photographs – the real missing photographs – was sent to the back of his mind. Hannah Brindley survived that night. She was alive and well – for how long, it seemed, all depended on Cam and what he chose to do next.

'Then we need a serious talk,' Cam said.

Tabernacle looked out at the pub again. When he spoke, a quiet resignation had drifted into his voice. 'I think you should get cleaned up, and I should have a beer. Maybe something stronger.' Cam nodded. His plan had worked. That said, if lathering Tabernacle in peanut butter would get him talking, he would have agreed to that too.

As soon as they were inside the old, converted coach house, crossing under the aged wooden beams overhead, Tabernacle headed to the bar, while Cam went through the back for the gents and the sinks. He gave himself a full cat's lick with soap from the dispenser, even running it through his hair. The cuts and abrasions stung, but nowhere near as much as the pain beneath the skin. This was fifteen championship rounds with an unbeaten heavyweight level of old-school pain — the kind you used to get at school or in training to toughen you up. It had been a while since he'd taken beatings the likes of the one he'd received in fits and starts these last few days. And yet, he somehow felt more alive than ever.

He emerged from the bar to see that, as predicted, Nala hadn't left Tabernacle's side. She obviously thought he might be hoarding some secret pork products on his person. In front of Tabernacle, at a booth overlooking the early afternoon clouds, sat two pints of ale. Before Cam could say anything, Tabernacle put a hand up.

'If you don't want the ale, I'll have it,' he said. 'It just didn't feel right, not buying you a pint after you'd come to fetch me and all.'

Cam joined him. Tabernacle appeared almost relaxed, and Cam realised that whatever the ramifications of his revelations, lifting the weight of them after so many years must be quite the relief. Even if it did mean the weight of the authorities coming down on him instead.

Cam took the pint and had a foamy sip. 'So, Jess Tabernacle is actually Hannah Brindley,' he said.

Tabernacle blew out hard. 'It's true,' he replied. His eyes were bright again, like when he'd been wielding that stripper pole only an hour earlier. 'She has to be.'

'You don't know for sure?'

'I mean, I do know it's her. But it's not the kind of thing you go and ask for a DNA test about.'

Cam leant forward, unable to keep his curiosity at bay. 'Tell me everything.'

Tabernacle had a glance around and decided that the coast was clear enough to speak — and when he did speak, he went on for approximately thirty minutes. He only broke off to buy himself two more beers, during which time, Cam had barely made it a quarter of the way down his own glass.

Tabernacle told a desperately sad and near-impossible story. How one night, prompted by a disturbance on Hickling Broad, he'd found a young girl in the woods, wandering drenched and alone, in a pretty party dress, holding a little stuffed dog. No sign of any parents in sight. She was catatonic, unable to speak, and carried a look so far away, Tabernacle had thought she might never come back to the present. Cam lost count of the amount of times Tabernacle said, 'It was the eighties, it was a totally different time', as he told Cam how he had taken the girl home to his cottage and shown the child to his wife.

His wife, Glynnis, was overwhelmed and immediately besotted with the child, and wrapped her up gently in a blanket, crying tears of joy as she began to settle – although Hannah's gaze never lost that unfathomable distance, and she seemed to slip deeper into a catatonic state. For the first few days, she simply couldn't be reached.

After a few weeks though, she showed signs of outward understanding, and even small patches of relief as she spent more time in the care of Mr and Mrs Tabernacle. Glynnis had believed that the child was some sort of gift from the heavens, a last-ditch reward for living a good life devoid of complaining that they themselves hadn't been able to bear children. Tabernacle had had no idea how to tell his wife that the child couldn't stay with them forever – but the child seemed to grow stronger with them, and grew into their routine.

The Tabernacles lived a supremely insular life. Glynnis never left the house on account of a chronic case of gout. She existed largely in a chair in the front room, the one Johnjo now favoured in tribute, only read romance novels, and watched soaps and the classic movies Johnjo loved. She had no care for the outside world, a hangover from the Second World War's decimating grip on her parents, which had been passed down to her. She believed the news was only ever bad, so she ignored it. Which meant that there were no newspapers at home, no news programmes on the television, no bulletins on the radio. The result? Glynnis was completely unaware that a family had gone missing at all.

Johnjo, however, as someone known in the community, visited his local pub often and heard the story of the missing Brindley family. It took so long, because nobody knew they were missing — Freddie Brindley worked for himself, and his children's absences from school were not uncommon. It was on the cleaner's fourth weekly visit to Brindley Hall that she realised they weren't just out for the day … for the fourth week in a row. Word spread, the news media cranked up, and Johnjo went to the newsagents to read the story for himself. There, on the front of the *Eastern Daily Gazette*, was a picture of the child who now lived with them.

Like that, it was utterly incontrovertible. The girl that they had begun to call Jess was, without doubt, Hannah Brindley. The daughter of the socialite couple who had gone missing.

Johnjo's heart broke, and he never showed Glynnis the newspaper. She was a fragile woman who he loved without compromise, and she was head over heels for the girl. Johnjo too, had grown an abundant devotion to Jess, and he battled with himself what to do. He often wondered what he'd do if the girl's parents returned, and truthfully felt he had no idea. He was just lucky that it never happened. And even more lucky that none of the search parties nor authorities thought to directly ask the old Norfolk boy and his wife in the little thatched cottage if they'd seen anything. He felt they were all lucky, the girl included.

He knew of the Brindleys and their flashy ways – never out of the papers, often causing a ruckus locally with some show-off scheme or other. Tabernacle was convinced that he and his wife would take better care of the girl than her real parents ever had – and far better than any foster system at the time, which was the reality of what he would be giving her back to with the parents still missing. With them, Jess would have love in endless quantities and a guaranteed roof over her head for as long as she lived.

And so, a difficult decision was made. Johnjo kept waiting for her to remember something about her old life and ask questions, but she never did. Glynnis kept her close and homeschooled her. It was only in her mid-teens when Jess ventured out into the world and really saw society for the first time, and if ever anyone asked; they were fostering her. Jess had grown up under the assumption that she'd been adopted young and had never pursued her birth parents. As a teen, whatever rebellious streak that arrived in her manifested itself in begrudging the parents that gave her up. She didn't remember them, nor anything prior to her life as a Tabernacle. Or, as Johnjo put it, she refused to remember. And so, the small villages of North Norfolk didn't seem to bat an eyelid; any connection between Jess and Hannah Brindley never made. It was a weird upbringing, but one that Tabernacle was sure had served her better than the alternative.

'As far as I am concerned,' Tabernacle said finally, with firmness, 'that girl is my daughter and always will be.'

Cam leaned back in his seat and blew out hard. It was mind-blowing, what had happened here. Not just that the

Tabernacles had got away with it, but that it had never been picked up – not by anybody.

'You … I mean, how didn't you report this? This girl … she could have been anyone's child and you … kidnapped her!'

Tabernacle shot a stony look at him. 'We saved her.'

'She wasn't your child to save.'

Tabernacle stared at him, daring Cam to push more. Eventually, he softened, and a mist cast over his eyes. 'She was a gift. She was given to us. We couldn't have children of our own, and Glynnis… This was a gift from God. And you didn't argue with my Glynnis when it came to God. She deserved this. And that girl deserved love.'

Cam could only blow out another breath. Through the shock of revelation, he could see clearly that the Tabernacles had almost – through the abrupt joy of finding this child – brainwashed themselves into thinking they were doing something good.

'You don't really collect newspapers, do you?' was all he could say.

'Do I bollocks,' said Johnjo. 'But those … those seemed important.'

Cam could understand the Tabernacles' actions to an extent, but felt that they had crucially overlooked what the truth might mean to Jess now she was an adult.

'She is in her mid-forties,' said Cam.

'I know.'

More than the fleeting buzzes of what he now had to admit was attraction, Cam felt connected to Jess Tabernacle, Hannah Brindley, whatever the hell she was going to be called now, in much deeper ways. They were similar spirits, both carrying pasts that, for whatever reasons, they couldn't confront – no matter how much they still defined them.

'This can't go on forever,' Cam said. 'You know that – don't you?'

Tabernacle thought hard on this and looked out at the rolling water of the river. The early afternoon had brought with it a bright sunlight that fought hard for prominence against the grey sky. In front of them, on the other side of the small road that separated the pub from the water, sat a herd of picnic tables, all empty. The scene was serene, peaceful. But like so many places, during so many moments in history, real horrors lingered beneath the waterline, ready to break through the surface tension when you least expected.

The old man smiled softly. 'I always knew the day would come that I would have to answer for this. Although I'll confess, a large part of me hoped I'd be dead by that time.'

'You have to tell her,' said Cam.

Tabernacle tried to say something but found he couldn't. He oiled his palate with ale and tried again. 'This has gone on for so long now, I worry about what it might do to her.'

About time, thought Cam. 'Never mind what it might do to her,' he said. 'She's an adult who deserves the truth. Don't take this the wrong way, but I can't believe you've gotten away with it for so long. She never once asked you a question about the early years of her life? Nobody ever questioned who the girl was who suddenly lived with you?'

'I don't know where you've been in your life, Cam, but I've only ever been here. And life here turns slowly and quietly, one bend of the river at a time. It really wasn't as difficult as you might think. She was homeschooled, then gradually started stepping out into the world the older she got. She was showered with love at home, more than she'd ever known, clearly, and that seemed to be enough for her.'

'Maybe so, but it's all going to come out now. I don't just mean the authorities and the press – Jesus, the press will *love* this – but Jess, too. And when she knows the truth, she might not feel the way you hope she'll feel.'

Tabernacle jutted his bottom lip out, then pursed his mouth. Like he was struggling to chew the quandary. 'Yes, I'm aware.'

'I'm not going to lie to her,' said Cam, as he looked Tabernacle square. 'I'm an instruction manual, a walking case study of what the past can do to a person in the present. If this ever comes up, I'm going to tell her, because the truth is the most important thing for people in our positions to hear – because it's something concrete we can work from.'

Tabernacle looked at Cam, and the first crack in his defiance started to appear. He spoke with his eyes turned down to the polished wood of the table. 'If anything, it would be easier if it came from you. All of it.'

'You don't get out of it that easy,' Cam countered firmly. 'She has to ask me those questions first. But it's the truth she's going to get from me. And it's the truth she should get from you too.'

Tabernacle nodded once and got back to his ale. 'That's all I would hope for too.'

Cam looked at the man who was resigned to risking the girl he had called his daughter for almost forty years. Was forty years of having a daughter worth it to see it all spoiled by some well-intentioned duplicity at the very start?

Cam didn't know the answer to that, but he was sure Tabernacle was going to find out the answer for himself soon enough.

A thought struck Cam while the cogs were turning. 'Johnjo, did you ever see anything of the rest of the family?

They're all still missing too, but maybe they're not dead. Like Jess?'

Johnjo shook his head. 'I only ever saw Jess. I have no idea about any of the others and didn't know to look for them at the time. As I say, the Brindley story came later. If I'd known about the boy... Well, I'm sorry I didn't.'

Then how did she get out? Cam wondered. If the car went into the water that night, how could Hannah – the smallest, youngest and most vulnerable of the lot – have been the only one that survived? If they all got out, what could possibly make two parents and a devoted brother leave her behind?

Cam found that he wanted to leave. Tabernacle, seemingly needing some space himself, said that he could make his own way home. Cam got up, whistled to Nala, and stood by the table. 'We've probably still got time before that club opens and Travis and his thugs are found,' he said, not quite able to look the man in the eye. These revelations were just so ... stunning. He needed time to figure out where his own head and heart lay. 'Stay here. I'll go and fetch Jess, and we can work out what to do next.'

Tabernacle just nodded and looked back out of the window at the river, a man seeing his past, present and future hang over destruction by a thread. All he could do now was sit back, sip Norfolk ale, and wait to face the music, whatever tune it played.

42

Hitting the road once more didn't do much good for Cam. If anything, the constant movement only made him feel even more like he was on the run.

With Nala back in the passenger seat, he rolled out of Horning village back up Main Street, his head swimming helplessly. Not only was the Jess Tabernacle/Hannah Brindley revelation earth-shattering, but another big question had grown so much in volume he couldn't do anything to drown it out. What was the real reason the corrupt Lord Chalmers and the aged gangster Tyrone Travis were so hell-bent on keeping this a secret? They must be responsible in some way for what happened to them – but why had they done it? Why make this family disappear?

And what had Travis had meant about 'the real pictures'?

There was another set of photographs out there.

Was this what they had killed for?

If not, why else would they want to keep this matter secret?

Travis himself had said that he was fond of 'losing' bodies around the Great Yarmouth coastline – had he done the same with the Brindleys, minus Jess? Is that why the three had never been found? Were they quite literally lost at sea? But if that were the case, and Travis, or Chalmers, or both, had murdered the Brindley family, why was Jess excluded? What gave her a free pass? Had she alone managed to escape them?

And if this line of thought was true, the biggest question of all loomed overhead: why was it necessary for the Brindleys to die at all?

To answer that, Cam had to find out what had gone wrong in the relationship between the men. He remembered an old Indian saying he'd learned while stationed in Hyderabad for a while.

Zan zar zameen.

An old Pashto proverb which stated what men were supposed to fight for and honour at all costs – and was consequently the root cause of so many murders. *Women, gold, land.*

Brindley was a financial advisor, who looked after people's money for a living. A massive motivator for murder was sitting right there in his job description.

Cam's phone rang and he answered, the voice filling the car.

'Hello?'

'Cam? It's Rogers here,' the familiar voice said in a breathless patter. 'Can we meet? I've got the results back from the computer. As I guessed, those boys down in the tech department thought it was Christmas when I brought that thing in, they couldn't wait to get tinkering on it. Next time I need them to expedite a case, I'll bring it stuck in a vintage Gameboy and see if that does the same trick. But they've copied the drive and I've got what was on there. I need to speak to you about it.'

Cam hadn't expected such speed and was pleased. Hotel Wroxham was just ahead and he needed to pick up his things from there anyway. He didn't want to stay long – that club would open, and those men would surely be back there to look for him – but maybe he could ask his new friend Darwin for some discretion. It would have to be quick. He turned left after the department store's McDonald's, then right between the fishing tackle shop and the toy store.

'I've gone back to the hotel, could you meet me there? I'll make sure we've got some privacy.'

'Give me twenty minutes,' said Rogers. She hung up while Cam was parking. This would be fine, he thought, because it would give him time to find Jess beforehand. He picked a spot just along from where he'd parked earlier, easily identifiable thanks to the vehicle's outline still etched in glass shards on the concrete. He'd have to get some mobile repairs done on the van soon enough. It wasn't the most subtle of transportations and the police might pull him over. Nevertheless, that was for another time.

He killed the ignition near the hedges by the river, then hopped out and started running. Anyone could be watching, and it sent the nape of Cam's neck abuzz. He wouldn't admit it, but deep down he'd have loved to hop straight in a warm bath with a snorkel and hide the rest of the afternoon away in his porcelain womb. But that wasn't going to solve a damn thing, apart from his growing headache.

As the afternoon had worn on, the sun had tilted westerly and a stubborn, biting chill had kicked up. He zipped up the dryrobe tight to his chin as he headed across the road to the department store. He dropped through his favourite clothing section to the food court, a purposeful pace to his step. He headed for the fruit.

Cam couldn't see her. He walked along the rows, checking down each one as he went. By the time he got to the dairy aisle at the far end of the building, he still hadn't found Jess. He walked over to a staff member who was wrestling a box of red wine onto a shelf. She was wearing a red jumper emblazoned with the name of the department store on the breast, just like the one Jess had worn the previous day.

'Excuse me,' he said. 'Is Jess Tabernacle working today? Is she about?'

The woman looked at him with a mixture of intrigue and contempt, glancing him up and down as if to see whether he was worthy of an answer. She apparently decided that he might be. 'She was in this morning, but I haven't seen her since lunch. Might have gone home sick, but I dunno.'

Strange. And unsettling. Cam thanked her and went to the checkout. She wasn't there either and he felt a growing frustration. It didn't take him long to canvass the whole place and determine she was nowhere to be seen. More than that, everyone he asked hadn't seen her that day either.

Agitated, he took out his phone and called Tabernacle's home number.

He waited, listening to the dial tone in hope, but nobody answered.

He then dialled the pub.

'Hello, the Heron's Reach?' A friendly voice answered.

'Hi, I'm trying to find a friend of mine, Johnjo Tabernacle? He's an older man, I was in having a drink with him earlier – is there still a guy by the riverside window, ploughing his way through pint after pint of Southwold bitter?'

The line went dead for a moment before the voice came back on. 'Yep, he's really tied one on, has this fella.'

'And is he alone?' he asked.

'Oh yes,' the voice replied. 'It's a solitary kind of drink, the one he's on.' Cam offered thanks and hung up.

Jess wasn't with her father, and she wasn't in work.

He didn't know enough about her to think where else she might be. He had no idea what her life away from her father and her work actually entailed. She'd gleefully told Cam only yesterday that it was either work or home for her in terms of interests. But given the scale of what he'd only recently learned about who she really was, how pivotal she could be if that information got into the wrong hands, it concerned him.

Where on earth was she?

43

In the lobby, Darwin was once again at his post. As soon as he saw Cam, he stood and held his hands up. 'I saw what happened to your vehicle, Cam. I'm very sorry about that, but I do feel compelled to tell you that according to hotel policy, vehicles are left in the car park at the owner's own risk.'

Cam couldn't help smiling.

'Don't worry, Darwin, I'm not the litigious type,' he said. 'Look, I'm sorry to ask this, but would you mind if I switched rooms again?'

Darwin breathed a sigh of relief, then transformed his demeanour to that of the consummately concerned concierge. 'There's something wrong with your suite?'

'No, not at all, it's just that everyone seems to be able to find me and I'd rather not have the hassle. If anyone asks for me, please could we keep it just between us?' Cam slid a ten-pound note across the desk with a wink. Darwin picked up a newspaper from his side of the desk and placed it on the note.

'Of course, Cam,' he said, lifting the newspaper back to its original start point. Cam looked down to see the note was gone.

'Is there anything else I can do for you?' the paid-off receptionist asked.

'Yes, please,' said Cam, and he leaned in conspiratorially. 'I've got someone over for a meeting very soon. Is there anywhere quiet, perhaps, that we could sit and have a chat? Not the bar or restaurant please this time, not after the disturbance from a certain Lord this morning.' Cam smiled softly, to let him know that they were now teammates in Cam's discreet escapade.

Darwin smiled in response. 'Of course, Cam – I felt so let down by his behaviour.' Cam thought it would be fun to really piss on Darwin's perception of Chalmers by telling him a few other choice details, but thought better of it. 'The snooker room isn't booked,' Darwin continued. 'Why don't you pop in there, and I'll run and get you some refreshments myself.'

'That sounds ideal.'

Darwin beamed. 'It's just the right-hand door by the men's toilets. If you go in there, I'll keep it booked out as long as you need. Would you care for something while you wait?'

'A coffee would be just fabulous.'

Darwin stood. 'Of course. And I'll see if we can get that doggie full English to make up for what this little one missed in the morning.' He nodded down at Nala.

'Now you're talking,' said Cam. He thanked Darwin then retreated to find the door to the snooker room.

It was an archetypal billiard room, the kind that you would find on vintage daytime murder mysteries and in stately homes all around the country. It seemed almost lifeless without the thick fog of smoke that had so clearly been a feature for most of its existence; nicotine stains ran down the walls. It appeared that this room was the only one in the whole hotel that hadn't yet seen a renovator's touch.

The billiard table itself had no balls in any of the pockets, nor any cues in the rack on the side, the vast green felt now serving as a huge conversation starter and very little else. Cam, feeling that when Darwin said it hadn't been booked out, he'd missed the suffix 'since 1980', walked past the table, Nala at his heels, and took a seat at one of two coffee tables on the end.

He waited. It was cool and quiet, and – in an act of sense rare to him in recent days – he started his breathing exercises while he had a minute. He didn't want to rush to the conclusion that Jess was categorically missing but ... he didn't like the coincidence that he couldn't reach her.

In for three.

Hold for five.

Out for eight.

Just a little calming top-up to keep straight.

Nala hopped into his lap but jumped off again as soon as Darwin reappeared. He carried a coffee as promised, and a tin bowl that looked like it had been filled with cat vomit, which Nala immediately started to wolf down.

'She makes friends everywhere we go, this one,' Cam said, then nodded to the bowl. 'That's a full English?'

'The very freshest,' Darwin said, quickly fussing over her before leaving. It didn't take long after that for Rogers to arrive. She walked in with an urgent, harried air, folding an umbrella. A shower must have swept by overhead.

'Well, this is ... unique,' Rogers said, as she pulled out a file, her movements charged, energised. She was either under extreme pressure, Cam thought, or excited to show him something. Maybe even both.

'Everything feels unique at the moment,' he said.

'It's a trait that's going to continue I'm afraid,' said Rogers, taking a sheaf of printouts from the file. She handed the top one to Cam. It was a spreadsheet with all manner of names and numbers, in an array that he found immediately indecipherable.

'I'm not a numbers guy,' he said. 'What am I looking at?'

'This is an account overview. Or moreover, an overview of Brindley's wealth management portfolio. That's a list of his clients, and on the right there, the funds invested, where they were invested, and the value at the far end.'

'Talk me through it,' said Cam, excited to the point of impatience.

'OK, so all the names that we came up with from those photos correspond to names in the database. They were all Brindley's famous clients, including of course, names that weren't represented by photographs.'

Cam looked at the names and scanned through them. True enough, those famous surnames were represented, mixed in with a lot of other names he hadn't seen before. One name wasn't there however: Tyrone Travis.

Rogers pressed on.

'You can see their initial investments when they started working with Brindley, on the left, with all the investment vehicles they put money into as we go across to the right.' Cam was just about following it and was using the name Chalmers as an example.

In the row next to Chalmers' name, the figure £264,000 sat in the initial investment column. In the columns along that same row were names of things that sounded either important, high-tech or just plain nonsense. By Rogers' logic and instruction, those funds had been used to invest in things called WorldCo Ltd, Standardised Securities, and FlowBox LLC.

'The final column is the valuation of the portfolio,' said Rogers, 'as of the tenth of November 1987.'

Rogers looked at Cam with raw excitement. And Cam felt a puzzle piece drop.

'The day they went missing,' he said.

'Spot on. And if you look at those numbers in that column? What can you see?'

Cam did as he was told and saw a pattern emerging immediately. It didn't take a degree in accounting to work out that every single person on this list had invested heavily, and by the tenth of November, the portfolios were greatly reduced in value.

Chalmers original £264,000 had reduced to just £15,000.

Others had gone from £390,000 down to just over £40,000. £70,000 down to £5,000.

It was a financial disaster. A portfolio of investment shame.

Rogers approached the snooker table and laid out printouts, one after the other, on the green baize. Cam joined her and switched on the overhead snooker light. Each piece of paper lit up bright white against the verdant felt.

'These are portfolio overviews of each and every client.' Rogers said. 'The data is represented as graphs of performance. Do I need to tell you what's going on here?'

Cam looked across all the graphs, over twenty of them, and watched the same pattern replicated on each chart. Each portfolio began with an excellent start, with overwhelming positivity across the gamut of examples Cam could see. Each then adopted a strong rising curve, reaching new heights, before an obvious disaster had struck them all – because near the end of each graph's timeframe, every portfolio imploded, the line plunged, and value plummeted to almost zero.

He looked at the date. During October 1987, each and every investment these people had made under Freddie Brindley's watch had been reduced to almost nothing.

Zan Zar Zameen, Cam thought. *Gold.* On these pages was a hell of a lot of motive.

'Mid-October, the whole thing turns into a disaster,' said Cam. Rogers pointed at the nearest graph, tracing the progress along the staccato line with her finger.

'Investments all big and strong,' she said. 'Years and months of growth, steady and rising. Then suddenly we get to October 1987 and it all goes wrong.'

'Black Monday,' Cam said. Rogers turned to look at him with surprise. 'I remember it from history lessons, because it sounded like an album the Smiths might release – and in high school, I flipping loved the Smiths.'

Rogers smiled with appreciation. 'Nineteenth of October 1987,' she said. 'Freddie Brindley had been using his clients' money to pour millions into US stock. But the funds Brindley was investing in were run via an automated program that had a unique unchecked failsafe – namely that if they suddenly dipped in value, stock was sold automatically. But at a fraction of its true value, leaving a massive loss. Everything was there one day, gone the next. Quite literally.'

'Chalmers lost everything,' Cam breathed.

'Pretty much,' replied Rogers. 'Brindley was never to know it would happen. Nobody knew. Experts didn't predict it, never mind an advisor like Brindley.'

'So … was Brindley killed as punishment for losing so much money?'

'Maybe,' Rogers replied, smoothing her long plait over her shoulder. 'We don't know. These numbers don't confirm that any of the people on this list are killers. Killing a whole family … that's a seriously dark business. And it wouldn't have done anything to get the money back.'

'Would a man like Tyrone Travis be capable of such a thing?' Cam asked.

Rogers looked perplexed. 'How the hell have you come across that name?'

'I met him this afternoon – he threatened me, Tabernacle and Tabernacle's daughter Jess, with all sorts if we didn't bring him the real photographs.'

Rogers was stunned, and Cam saw a hint of disapproval cross her face as she said, 'So that's where you were going when you came to fetch them.'

'Yep. But they were useless – Travis saw them and said they weren't the ones Chalmers was looking for.'

Rogers held up the first finger of each hand and drew them together. 'So Chalmers and Travis—'

'Are in on this together,' Cam finished.

'Jesus.' Rogers grabbed the sheet with the list of names. 'But he isn't on this list of clients.'

'I saw. He could have been using a pseudonym though.'

Rogers shook her head and leaned her hip against the snooker table. 'He's a loan shark, or at least he was. I wouldn't have thought investment was his style.'

Cam thought about that and conceded that she was probably right.

'Maybe. Was he on the guest list for the party?'

'No, he wasn't. That's a name I'd definitely remember. It doesn't mean he wasn't there though.'

'He's definitely involved – and he looked prepared to kill for it earlier.' The Gurkha's kukri jumped into Cam's mind, cruel and intimidating. 'What about the rest of the guest list. Do they match the client list here?'

Rogers shook her head. 'No. Well, some names appear on both, I should say, but most don't. It makes sense that Freddie would go to a glamorous party and run into a few of his famous friends by coincidence. And let's not forget, Travis is on neither.'

'Let's also not forget that Chalmers, however, *is*.'

'True.'

Rogers sighed. 'There's one more name on that list.'

'Who?' Cam asked.

Rogers shook her head. The news seemed to sadden her so much her usual spark was dimmed. 'A man called Gary Hilton.'

'Who's he?'

'He's the very man who told me the case was closed.'

Cam's eyes widened. Surely not. 'Your…'

'My chief.'

Cam could see how furious and betrayed Rogers looked. As if she'd come to accept the knife in her back, even though it still really, damn hurt. He didn't say anything, but knew the truth. This explained so much, especially about how the police had handled the matter. The dice were weighted from day one.

The revelations sat thicker than any smoke the room had ever experienced.

'Could someone on this list,' asked Cam, his mind a whirr, 'have employed Travis to put pressure on the Brindleys? Maybe it went wrong?'

'That's certainly a logical thought,' said Rogers.

Cam sighed. 'There's also something else I need to tell you. Something I think you need to take a seat for.' Her jaw sagged lower with every sentence as Cam made the decision. He told her the story of Jess Tabernacle – and how she was at that moment, missing.

November 1987

There is something the matter with Tommy.

I can't completely work it out. He seems distant, as if he's got one eye out of the window all the time, even though there isn't a window there. He seems like a bit of his brain is somewhere else.

He's had to have a couple of days off school. I don't really understand why. Mum says he's ill but he's not been throwing up and he's not got a temperature.

I'm trying to make him feel better, so I'm on my way upstairs with his favourite things. A Panda Pop, some marmalade toast and a copy of the *Beano* that arrived this morning. I managed to sneak the comic away before he could see it, because it was all part of my big surprise for him.

I carry these items up the stairs and when I get to the top, I listen out for him. The whole house is silent. In fact, the whole house has been quiet for days, ever since that party the other night. Ever since Mum came down the stairs with those weird men, nothing has been the same. We left right after that and when we got home, Mum and Dad went straight to their bedroom, leaving me and Tommy to do our teeth and put our pyjamas on.

After a while, Dad came out of their bedroom. I saw him through the kitchen window, sitting at the back porch, staring over the lake. I've barely seen Mum since, although she's been in and out of her bedroom for food. I think she must be poorly too.

Maybe there's something going around. Dad's been doing the school runs. He doesn't seem too affected, and he's working lots of hours just like normal. He says there's another party to go to on Saturday, and after all those times wishing I could go, I'm really hoping we can miss it.

I stand outside Tommy's room juggling the tray. It sounds quiet in there too. I manage to knock with my big toe at the bottom of the door but it's not very loud, so I shout: 'Tommy?'

When he answers, his voice sounds worlds away. 'Yeah?'

'Can I come in?' I ask.

'Give me a second,' he replies, and I stand there like a lemon for half a minute. 'OK,' he eventually calls.

I go in to find that his curtains are closed, and his room has become a dark cave. No wonder he's in a funny mood, sitting in here all day.

'I brought you some bits to make you feel better,' I say, and put the tray on his bed. He is sat at the little colouring station by the window that Mum made for him, but his colours are all packed away and his desk is empty.

He looks sheepish, like he's been caught doing something he shouldn't.

'Thanks, sis,' he says. His smile looks so pretend, it hurts my tummy.

'What are you doing?' I ask.

284

He looks like he doesn't know how to answer. He actually looks like he doesn't have any words in his head at all, like whatever words he might find wouldn't be enough. Like the stubborn little sister Mum says I am, I just stare at him till he decides to talk.

'I found something this morning,' he says. 'But you can't tell anybody about it. Not Mum. Not Dad. I think it would upset them all, if they saw it. So, I'm keeping it safe for them. I think if I hide what I found, it might go away.'

He's looking at the floor when he says this, as if he is trying to explain the situation to himself as much as to me.

'What did you find?' I ask.

He reaches into the little drawer of his colouring desk and pulls out a small yellow and red folder. I recognise it as the kind of flappy envelope photos come in when Mum gets pictures developed at the pharmacy. I reach for it.

'No!' he says, holding it tight to his chest like a favourite teddy.

'Where did you find them?'

'I came downstairs to get my comic but it wasn't on the porch, so I went into Dad's office to see if he'd accidentally taken it in there with him when he picked up the papers. He wasn't there but these were on his desk.'

'Are they pictures?' I ask.

'Yes,' Tommy says, and his eyes filled with tears. 'I don't really know what they are about, but no one should ever see them.'

44

Rogers stared at Cam in the dim light, her eyes piercing and still, and blew out as soon as he finished speaking. 'Hannah Brindley *survived*? She's been living as Jess Tabernacle all this time? This changes absolutely fucking everything,' she said. The wind had been so knocked out of her, she practically deflated into the chair.

'She survived...' Rogers repeated, and Cam could practically see the gears turning in her mind. 'She might know exactly what happened that night.'

Cam nodded slowly. 'But we have to be careful,' he said. 'Going too hard at her could cause so much damage. It might close her up for good.'

'Cam, I know of your history, and can certainly understand your sensitivity towards this girl and her issues...'

Cam felt a gust of rage at Rogers' use of the word 'issues'. It was this sort of thing, this sort of judgement, that put paid to any real progress in understanding the kind of problems Cam lived with. But so many people would never understand, Cam reminded himself, and cover-all phrases like 'issues' would have to do; he let the flame puff out.

Rogers continued. 'But she might have vital information that could change the entire landscape here. She might be able to put those responsible for her parents' disappearance away. She needs to be questioned.'

Cam thought about it and shook his head. 'I understand that, but if we can't approach this with care, the memories might cause a lot of damage to her.' That and the fact he didn't know where she was and couldn't direct Rogers to her if he tried.

Rogers looked like she wanted to counter that argument but thought better of it. Cam decided to keep her mind moving forward rather than in stasis on a thorny topic.

'What's the next move?' He asked.

'I take this lot back and try to build a robust team that won't be influenced by higher-ups or outside knobheads with cash,' she said. 'And then we build an ironclad case to prove Chalmers and Travis were involved in the Brindley disappearance. And their efforts to keep it quiet.'

'I'll provide statements asserting everything that happened to me, including who did it and when.' The only thing he was unsure of, was sharing the Tabernacles' duplicity in taking Jess/Hannah in. He had no idea, morally, how he wanted to handle that.

Rogers looked at him with admiration and smiled. 'You really have blown everything apart, you mad, stubborn bastard.'

Cam smiled as Rogers grabbed her things and headed to the door – but she paused with her hand on the handle. 'Just one more thing that's been nagging me,' she said, and looked at him with eyes downturned with melancholy. 'Tommy, the Tommy I knew, he would never – ever – have left his sister alone out there. He would have done anything for that girl. *Anything.*'

'What are you saying?'

She looked at him sternly and spoke with utter conviction. 'Now, then, whenever. That little boy I knew – he'd die for his sister. He would have done anything to get back to her. And the fact he hasn't after all this time… Well, it means that he either didn't know she survived, or he's dead. And that's hard to take.'

Cam nodded slowly as Rogers left.

Just … *breathe.*

He thought about what Rogers had just said to him, about blowing this case open at last. Cam felt the swell of people believing in him, and it was something that he'd not experienced for a long time. It caused pinpricks of tears to well in his eyes. Nala looked up at him from his lap, checking on him as always. He stroked the dog's head and kissed her on the spot between her eyes. 'Good girl.'

He thought of the rollercoaster ride of the last few days, the twists and turns, bumps and bruises. It had been a lot. And he thought about their plan to take Chalmers and Travis down. They'd need evidence, and although it was stacking up at last, so much of it was still circumstantial.

He needed something completely, undeniably incriminating.

Something Chalmers and Travis would do anything to keep quiet.

Something like those missing photographs. The *real* ones.

Where the hell were they? What did they show that was so important?

Whatever it was, they held the key. He was sure of it.

Cam hopped up, knowing what he needed to do, sure of where he was being drawn to, and went out into the lobby. On the front step, however, he paused. Nala looked at him with confusion at his stop–start antics. Should he run upstairs for more medication?

No, he thought. *No. I'm the master of this ship at the moment, and I'm doing fine.*

45

Cam found himself heading back to Hickling. There was something about the endlessness of the water there, and how every time he'd hit a dead end, the place had offered him direction. Hickling Broad, he was sure, held the key. This was where Hannah was found, same as the car. The answers had to be there.

He didn't care about the stares his van was getting anymore as he barrelled along the roads deep into Norfolk Broads national park. He just had to know what he was missing, and felt that the water, somehow, would show him the way – just like it had done countless times before.

He ran through the case in his head, urgently weaving questions and possibilities into something he hoped would finally make sense.

All four Brindleys had left the party that Saturday night in a car that ended up in the water. When that car was found, there were no Brindleys in it. More than that, Hannah Brindley had been alive all along – but Tabernacle found her soaked. She'd definitely been in the broad that night. She had survived in the frigid waters and went on to have another near-forty years of life – with or without an understanding of what had happened to her.

The parents, if they survived, would have gone back to Brindley Hall – or called the police. But what about the boy, Tommy? What had happened to him? If his body wasn't found, was he still alive somewhere too? Did he get out that night and end up lost, like young Hannah did? And if he did, where did he go?

Cam had a hunch that was bordering on supernatural that the answers would be found in Hickling. These waters were all cloaked in mystery, always harbouring myth. Whether it was oversized pike or tales of smugglers – there had to be something lingering in the eerie, mist-soaked ether of this near-mystical place.

As he got closer to the hulking body of water, the dark seemed to close in ever so slightly, and everywhere took on a violet tint. Driving in what felt like the country's most indiscreet vehicle, he did away with subtlety on approach and simply ploughed through the crime scene tape. He forged through the undergrowth, spitting mud in every direction, driving too fast – but he felt the pull so severely, his thirst for answers so strongly, he couldn't slow if he wanted to.

Before long, he was there, and parked at the clearing with an abrupt stop, the van skidding briefly before its weight managed to pause it. He wasted no time in jumping out, Nala joining him, now giddy, feeding off Cam's own determined energy. She sprinted into the water for a drink and after a few moments with her face to the surface, she cavorted along the lapping shoreline.

Cam, on the other hand, simply stood there, staring at that indigo sky and begged for answers.

He was convinced now, as he let the facts of the case wash over him, that the rest of the Brindleys had been murdered – or at the very least attacked and taken somewhere. Hannah surviving, Tommy's nature to protect his sister at all costs or even over his own body, Maud vanished from the face of the earth, Freddie in the thick of it with corrupt politicians and shady criminals – it all seemed to point that way. And he believed that Chalmers and Travis were responsible, while their collective motivations remained unclear.

Chalmers' personal motivations were crystal, considering how much money Brindley had lost him. But where did Travis fit in? He was a loan shark, lending money at exorbitant rates. Had Freddie Brindley borrowed from him? There was no evidence to support that.

It made no sense to Cam.

He looked around at the ground around him and tried to picture the terrain forty years ago. If it was anything like it was now, it would have been wild, unforgiving and dense. His research told him these banks hadn't changed in years, even less now the area was protected as part of the wetlands reserve.

He tried to imagine what it would've been like for Hannah Brindley that night, running through the trees and bushes and the pitch black, drifting ever closer to catatonia.

It would be, singularly, the most terrifying thing a young person could go through, Cam was sure of it.

He looked at the spot where he knew the car had been found, now on his third visit in as many days to this exact location. If she had come up from a sunken position, where would she have gone? And if Tommy had got out too, where had they headed?

Tommy.

As a flock of geese wheeled overhead with a thumping of wings that sounded like a hummingbird in his ear, Cam switched his attention to the boy. What if they'd come up, and had to split up? What if Tommy had gone for help, and got caught?

If Tommy was alive now, was he someone like Jess? Somebody he knew, somebody he had come across, and never made the link.

You're going mad, Cam, he thought to himself.

He was never going to leave his sister. So, what if he was still here? Somewhere on the wetlands preserve, lost where nobody could stumble across him. The sadness of the thought threatened to drown Cam.

He imagined a scenario in which both children escaped the car. If they had come up here, and there was commotion on the bank as people sent them into the water, they may have swum somewhere else to get out, and emerged from the water where it was quieter. Cam whistled to Nala and started walking through the thick underbrush, past the nose of his van, and past where Chalmers had been hiding in the trees the other night.

The track disintegrated immediately, submitting to being choked and suffocated by tangled knots of trees that had grown with a determined abandon.

With the careful approach of a surgeon, Cam picked and plotted his way through, and eventually made it round to the next bay of the broad. It wasn't much further along as the crow flew, but it gave him a different vantage point of the area. It let him see that on this side, the broad opened right out to show its immense belly across the middle. He felt sick at the thought, hell, even at the prospect of children stuck and alone here. It was so vast. So unforgiving.

On the far side of the shallow bay, about a hundred metres away, there was a small tower which had a wind vane on the top. It was a tired, wooden miniature windmill, with no building underneath, except for a faded white ladder leading to a tatty white cube on the top, which still possessed a couple of blades that rotated slowly in the soft wind.

It would give him the perfect view.

Cam checked his phone, but there were no messages to answer. Nothing from Rogers, nothing from Gupta and Ferris, nothing from Jess, nothing from Tabernacle. Just him, Nala, and the depths of the Brindley mystery.

Cam made his way to the tower, weaving this way and that between the branches and uneven root systems underfoot. It was about ten metres high, with a thin support beam at the top from which he could stand and get a brilliant view across the entire broad.

'Stay here, darling,' he said to Nala, who had run off to relieve herself on the other side of the ladder. He tested its sturdiness and began to climb.

Once he got to the top, the breeze was stronger with less tree cover, but the view was mesmerising. A huge, barely touched body of water in the middle of Broadland, doused in pink and purple hues as another day extinguished on its surface. He gazed in wonder and took in its majesty. Nobody ever talked about the beauty of the Norfolk Broads in terms that met with how he was feeling right that second.

He looked across the broad at places a child might pull themselves out of the water. If he had an idea as to where Hannah had managed to escape, it might hold clues to what happened to the rest of them.

He swung his neck around to the right and looked across the reeds and bullrushes, catching sight of a marsh harrier, cruising slowly, looking for one last meal of the day. It was an amazing creature, able through sheer force of muscle to almost float in place. He admired the fact that it expelled so much energy, simply to stay still. As he watched it, he turned to get a better view – and his right foot slipped.

Cam threw his arm out to the boxy wooden top of the tower and held onto it while he regained his footing. As he righted himself however, he heard something funny. It was a strange sound from the cube itself when he'd hit it.

He knocked on it. There was a soft, almost imperceptible echo within.

The square box was hollow.

It was about a metre square in size and there was a little hatch on the side.

He reached forward, took the handle and pulled it open.

Cam Killick had seen a lot of things in his time, some of the worst things humanly imaginable. Things that had scarred him for life and presumably still would in death.

But nothing, none of it, had prepared him for what was on the other side of that door.

November 1987

We left the party after only ten minutes.

It's at the same posh house on the edge of the big city, and the same posh things have happened. We'd been let out of the car by those men in funny suits, taken into the house to look at the buffet area, and offered a plate of cold meat and sausage rolls like it would keep us quiet. Mum and Dad both went upstairs this time.

I looked at Tommy and asked him. 'What do you think is happening?'

Tommy looked as glum as I'd ever seen him. 'I bet it's about those pictures,' he said.

'Where are they?' I asked in a whisper. The Pound Puppies are in my hand again and I worry I might rub their fur right off the way I stroke them.

'They're in my jacket pocket.' I looked at Tommy, then down at the pale blue sports jacket he was wearing.

'What have you got them here for?'

'I thought if I gave them back, things might get better.'

'Give them back to who?'

'The people who took them. But it won't work.'

'Why don't you just show them?' I said.

Tommy's eyes filled with fear. 'No. Promise me you won't mention it.' He took my hand, even putting the plate of sausage rolls down to do so. 'Promise me, Han.'

'I promise.' I'd do anything for Tommy.

Then there was shouting upstairs. A door slammed. Dad came downstairs, pulling Mum along behind him and they hurried us to put our plates down and go to the front door, where we had to wait a couple of minutes for our car to come round. When it did, someone started taking pictures, so we jumped in quickly and Dad drove off with a loud growl of the engine.

I turned to have a look out of the back window, and I could see the two men Mum and Dad had disappeared with. They were watching us go from the front steps while the person taking pictures continued to click away, the bright flash popping against the hedges of the garden.

I was glad we left those men. The one with the red face, and the one who looked like a big heron with legs too long for his body. I hope we never see them again. Now, me and Tommy just look out of the windows in the back of the Jaguar, watching the countryside eat the lights as we head back deep into the woods and rivers towards home.

After a little while of driving in the dark, there is a flash in Dad's mirror.

'Shit,' he says, and I don't think I've ever been more shocked. He said a rude word right in front of us. I suppose we'll get another present out of it, but I really don't care. I just want to go home.

We keep driving, trees all around us now, with no street-lights, and I keep sneaking glances behind – at the car that is now following us. Tommy does the same. His right leg won't stop shaking.

Not long after that, Mum screams.

Dad hits the brakes and we lurch to a sudden stop, which hurts my tummy through the seatbelt. Through the front window, I can see a black car is parked crossways between the trees. Blocking our way.

Suddenly, all the doors open at once. I look around for the other car, which has parked just behind us. Its doors are opening too, and people are getting out and surrounding us. They are big men. They have scary eyes.

Mum is breathing fast and shouting things I can't understand. Dad is shouting, too. 'Everyone stay calm, everyone stay quiet. I'll handle this, I promise, I will handle this.'

In fairy stories and kids' films, or at least the ones we've read and watched, daddies are like princes. They'll do anything, they might even *die* to protect the people that they love. I've seen them jump into volcanoes, fight huge trolls with swords, even in one very sad film, jump in front of a car so that their child didn't get hurt.

Our dad does none of that.

He does nothing.

Instead, he lets the people walk over and pull Mum out of the car, leaving me and Tommy in the back.

I can hear shouting outside. I'm frozen, I'm so scared.

They are arguing about something called blackmail, and pictures.

Where are the pictures?

Where are the photos?

I know where they are.

I look at Tommy and ask him the question – just with my eyes. *Please give them the pictures.*

He shakes his head. I know he thinks it will make it worse, but what could be worse than what's happening right now?

Dad is shouting. He doesn't have the pictures, he keeps saying, and Mum is screaming and crying too. I hadn't realised, but I'm doing the same. The heron man walks up to Dad and grabs him too roughly. Pulls him out of the car too.

A gun is put to his head, another thing I've seen from films.

I feel like I might faint. I squeeze the Pound Puppies so hard I wonder if their seams might pop.

The same man turns the steering wheel, and people behind are pushing our car forward. We are moving very slowly, but the engine is still turned off.

The car dips forward.

With a huge splash, water bounces over the bonnet, onto the windscreen. It forces the front doors shut. Dad is screaming outside. 'I don't have the pictures, I've never seen them! I let you have everything, everything we agreed.'

We're in deeper now. I can feel it. The car is beginning to float. Tommy is shouting, pulling at the door, screaming for help. I do the same, but I'm almost too scared for any sound to come out. I see water at my feet, gushing into the Jaguar, the lovely green carpet turning brown with mud.

Mum and Dad are in the water too now, screaming, but they can't come any closer because the gun is pointing at them.

The heron man is shouting: 'Your kids are sinking. You'd better give us those pictures.'

Tommy is next to me, doubled up in fear, his knees under his chin. He looks at me and shakes his head. 'They'll hurt Dad even more if they see what he's done.'

He will never give up those pictures.

I scramble to see through the windows, realising that the voice screaming for Mum and Dad is mine. Mum is screaming for us too, and one of those horrible men holds her by the hair. Dad has the gun to his head again, and the water is getting higher. We're drifting further out and further out, when Tommy speaks.

'Han, we have to go *now*.'

With more strength than I thought he had, Tommy manages to open the side door, just enough. Water pours in. I look out of the back window and see that all those people can't see us, because Tommy's side of the car is facing out towards the middle of the water now, not the bank. Tommy grabs me and pulls me with him. It's so tight, and the car is half under, but he pulls me through — and as soon as we're out, the door is sucked shut by the water. It sinks lower.

I once fell into our lake at home, but it was a summer's day and kind of fun. This water is freezing. My breathing is coming in tiny sparrow breaths, and my chest goes so tight it's like I'm being squeezed. I can't move my legs, I can't even scream even though every bit of me seems to want to, but Tommy keeps me afloat as he starts to swim.

I don't even have my water wings on.

I'm beginning to feel something different too, like everything that's happening is getting too big for my body. I'm more scared than I've ever been, but at the same time I'm beginning to feel not that scared at all. I *can't* feel it — just like my arms and legs.

Tommy is on his back, kicking hard, holding the back of my head onto his chest so that my face is looking at the stars. There's lots of them, and on another night, they would be beautiful. I can't feel my fingers anymore, and

I can't tell whether I'm holding onto the Pound Puppies. I try to squeeze just in case.

I tilt my head to try to see what's going on back towards the shore, and in the glare of headlights from the cars that stopped us, I can see Mum and Dad on their knees in the water. Dad is just looking at his Jaguar car – that now sinks with a plopping hiss out of sight.

We are paddling off away from Mum and Dad, but I can just about make out the guns that are still pointed at their heads.

The heron man takes Mum's hair again and pulls her up. He seems to show her to Dad, like a rabbit he's caught. There is a distant POP, and her screaming stops.

I'm going to be sick.

'Don't scream, Han,' Tommy whispers to me, through panting breaths.

I want my mum.

I want my mum.

She's there, but she's not.

She drops into the water. Dad is screaming now. It's Mum's real name he's saying. The one I don't think ever suited her. *Maud.*

The heron man walks to him now, the gun up.

I don't want to watch anymore.

I'm not sure I can look away.

I lie back and look at the stars again. I look at the moon. It's big and far away – where I want to be. Anywhere but here. I can feel myself drift. I'm going to space. Higher and higher. I can look down and see me and Tommy.

At last Tommy pulls me out of the water, into the trees and puts me on some grass. He leans me against a tree trunk and tells me he's going to get help. That he just needs to see where we are. He tells me it'll all be OK.

I think that's what he's saying.

I can't feel anything. I don't even feel the cold. I don't remember why I'm here.

I don't know who the boy running off into the bushes is.

I don't know why I'm holding a toy dog in my hand.

Where am I? Why am I so cold?

Who am I?

I don't know what I'm doing. I'm by myself. I'm terrified.

I get up and walk into the darkness.

46

Cam closed the door, leaving everything as he had found it – with one exception.

In the immediate aftermath of the sight, he found that life didn't feel the same way anymore. Everything was tainted.

Nala looked up at him from the bottom, and he found himself softly shaking his head at her. He took out his phone, stared at the horizon and dialled.

'Rogers?' he said. 'I know I've just seen you, but we need to meet immediately.'

'Christ, Cam,' the flustered detective said. 'What's happened now? I've only just got back to the nick.'

Cam checked his watch. 4:32 p.m. It was getting closer and closer to a time where workers might show up at Sirens, and free Travis. 'We need to find Jess Tabernacle immediately. And ... I ... we just need to meet now. Trust me.' Cam didn't know how to explain what he'd seen. Not yet. He thought about how the landscape had changed for good – and how he had to share it with not just Rogers, but Jess and Johnjo Tabernacle as well. Ferris and Gupta, too. 'The Heron's Reach in Horning, meet me there as soon as you can.'

Cam hung up and looked at the sky one last time.

Darkness was inching closer to full takeover, not just in the atmosphere, but in Cam's own heart too.

He climbed down and made his way carefully back to his van.

When Cam arrived at the Heron's Reach, Horning was dead and covered in cloud-packed darkness. He parked in the pay-and-display next to the *Southern Comfort*, the riverboat's lights on and hopeful, even though it was far too cold and late in the year to be doing evening trips. Maybe they were cleaning it.

'Be right back,' Cam said as Nala hunkered down in her dog bed.

He went around to the pub's front door, glancing inside the windows as he passed. In the amber glow of the little log fire, Cam saw Rogers was already there – as was Tabernacle. He went straight for their table. Tabernacle evidently hadn't stopped supping since Cam had left earlier that afternoon. His cheeks were ruddy as overripe tomatoes, and his eyes clouded with the drink. He merely tipped his glass in Cam's direction by way of a greeting.

Rogers, on the other hand, immediately stood and put her hand up to halt Cam from coming any nearer. She looked like the pressures of the case, and all its back-and-forths, were draining her.

'Has Jess turned up?' she asked. 'I went out to Tabernacle's but there was nobody there.'

'Not that I know of,' Cam replied. 'Johnjo, have you seen her?'

'Who?' said Tabernacle.

'Never mind.'

Cam's phone began to ring in his pocket. Filled with hope that it might be the missing woman, he pulled it out – only to find an unknown number on the screen. He looked at Rogers. The last thing he wanted to do was answer it, but Rogers said: 'It might be her.'

Cam lifted the handset to his ear.

'Killick,' said the voice. Cam's hackles raised. It was Chalmers, his voice unmistakable. Cam looked around, feeling the burn of observation on his neck, but the pub was quiet save for a couple of old ale hounds, tucked by the open fire.

'What do you want?' Cam said, his eyes roving.

'Having a pint?' Chalmers goaded. Cam's arms buzzed pins and needles right to his fingertips. 'Can I buy you one? And your friends too?'

Cam walked away from the table to look into the recesses of the pub, past the bar. He saw no one.

'Not in there,' Chalmers said. 'Why don't you come and have a drink. We can talk about how we can all resolve this.'

'Where do you suggest?' Cam asked.

'Look outside.'

Cam walked to the window and pressed his face close to the glass to avoid the reflection of the pub's interior. He couldn't see anything.

'On your right,' Chalmers said, and Cam peered along the river, back to the *Southern Comfort*'s lit windows – in one of which stood Chalmers with his arm raised. 'Don't worry, there's a fully licensed bar on here, so Mr Tabernacle can keep pickling himself.'

How had Chalmers found them? 'I'd rather not, thanks. Sorry if you've wasted a ticket.'

'That's a shame, there's someone here with me who'd love to see you.'

305

Cam thought about Chalmers' associates he'd met, and didn't like the idea of seeing any of them again one bit. 'Then I'm definitely not getting on.'

'A shame,' repeated Chalmers. 'I thought you'd be pleased to see who I've convinced to come along. Plus, it would be nice for her to see her dad.'

Jess.

Panic shot through him, his worst fears dragged to life.

Cam was hanging up and back at the table before Chalmers could say another word. 'We need to go, now,' he said.

'What do you mean?' Rogers asked, more than a little irritated.

Cam glanced at Tabernacle, who was looking up at Cam like he was a TV programme he was only half-interested in. Cam leaned in to Rogers and spoke in hushed tones. 'It's Chalmers, he wants a chat. On the boat outside. He's got Jess.'

Cam watched the information roll across Rogers. Her jaw set. 'We best get over there then,' she said. 'Come on, Johnjo.'

Tabernacle stood with the bovine gaze of a creature being herded, and they filed out into the night towards the grand steamboat. The motor was still running, and steam swelled off the engine block. Cam had never been on it, and if it weren't for the occasion he'd have liked to ask the pilot to take them for a spin. It was two-storeys high, clad in white paint with dark red and gold trim, and looked every inch the vintage specimen.

They crossed the gangplank onto its rear deck, and Rogers opened the door next to the roped-off rear stairs, holding it wide to allow Tabernacle and Cam to enter the cabin. The door closed, and it was impressively quiet considering the engine noise they'd just heard.

As he walked in, the sight Cam was greeted by filled his stomach with grease. Across a polished wood dance floor, was a bar. And behind that bar was a man fixing himself a drink. Lord Chalmers. He smiled Hollywood-style at them – and was noticeably alone.

'Where's Jess?' Cam demanded, looking around.

But suddenly they were moving.

The boat had set off, the floor lurching forward gently beneath their feet – while behind them, the rear door opened again.

They all turned to look, and with his nose covered in a patchwork of plasters, in walked Tyrone Travis.

'Gotcha,' he said.

47

Cam's blood ran white-hot and bubbling. His head wanted to split open like a watermelon, the horses were bolting, and he put his hands on the side of his head to hold it all together.

Travis walked past Rogers, straight up to Cam. He thrust a knife, the kukri that was longer than Cam's forearm, up towards him. 'I am going to peel you with this, mark my words,' he snarled.

Rogers stepped forward to intercept, when behind Travis the door opened again, bringing with it a blast of engine noise – and Jess Tabernacle. She was being pushed in by Travis's son, the big, bearded Danny. They had to have been up with the pilot the whole time.

Tabernacle, who had been a drunken bystander up to this point, sobered in an instant. 'Jess, are you all right?' he asked, his voice hard-edged. Jess look red-eyed, tired and beaten, still in her work outfit.

'Jess? You OK?' Cam echoed Tabernacle's question.

'I'm not sure,' Jess answered, and she finally met Cam's eyes. She looked mired in confusion, she was still in there. 'I'd love an answer or two, if anyone has any?'

Travis sneered with an ungodly level of venom. 'Bit of a reunion,' he said, 'not that I expected it. Phones.' He held out a black bin bag and paced over to Tabernacle. 'Now.'

Tabernacle took out his phone and tossed it into the bag with a crinkle of plastic. 'You, sir, are a real wanker,' he said stoutly.

'I'll remember that.' Travis smiled. 'The rest of you.'

Rogers, Jess and Cam all took out their phones. Cam glanced at the screen as the others put theirs in the bag first. It showed the preview of a message from Gupta and Ferris, in their ludicrously named WhatsApp group. It didn't show everything, but enough for him to get the gist. It was another puzzle piece falling into place. He dropped the phone into the bag, which Travis tossed out of the window, instantly lost to the black.

The old man looked back at Chalmers. 'Who would've thought it would come to this?'

Chalmers simply shrugged. He took a revolver from his jacket, placed it on the bar, and topped off his ale from the pump. Beyond him, through the cabin windows, Cam could see the lights of the Heron's Reach spin beyond the glass as the boat turned out into the river.

How on earth had he been so stupid as to get on this thing? Jess's well-being had been at the forefront of his split-decision, but still. In anger at himself, his senses frothed and his panic bloomed, but he was somehow able to hold them at bay.

The gun had completely changed the dynamics. A knife was close quarters. A gun? The threat to life was every-where and with everyone. It had triggered his combat mind, the mind he was slowly reclaiming, and he was already looking for exits and strategy.

'What is it you all want?' Cam asked, backing up slightly towards one of the windows so that he could see left and right either way along the cabin. He was dizzy, cerebrally adrift, but fought for focus.

Travis, Danny and Jess were towards the stern, while Chalmers was towards the bow. Johnjo Tabernacle and DS Rogers were next to Cam in the middle. The physical threat was all coming from Travis and Danny at the back of the boat, but Chalmers also had so much skin in the game – and the gun.

It did somewhat surprise Cam, therefore, when Chalmers answered.

'If this boat sank right now, with all of us on it, it would be problem solved,' he said. 'But that doesn't work out too well for me. And it seems that making threats to you, Killick, doesn't really make much of a difference.'

'I was always a stubborn sort,' Cam replied.

'Yes, well done,' Chalmers said. 'But when I popped up to Yarmouth and found these boys tied to a stripper pole, you kind of sealed your fate.'

Travis butted in, his anger far too much to remain holstered, and Cam snapped round to him. 'We're heading out because on the other side of that water is miles and miles of marshes. You put a body in there, it moves around for years, getting more and more covered up. You will never be found.' He turned to Jess. 'Or at least you won't be this time, *Hannah*.' He spat the name at Jess with malevolence.

Jess looked at Travis with pure hatred, but it broke almost immediately into a broad, blank canvas of expression.

Oh no, thought Cam. Chalmers tipped his glass and bared a toothsome grin. *How did they know?*

As if reading Cam's query telepathically, Chalmers tutted. 'I thought I showed you how far I could reach.

310

Once you found that car, you put everyone around you at risk – even those you'd only just met.' He tilted his pint glass at Johnjo. 'You should see what his doctor writes about him.' Then he tipped the ale at Rogers. 'And her marriage is up the swanny river, but she's too stubborn to give in and admit it's over.'

'You watch your mouth,' Rogers seethed.

'And you can imagine it didn't take long to find out that there is no real Jess Tabernacle. No birth certificate. And then … a seven-year-old appears in 1987, soon after another seven-year-old disappears? Hmm, ever wondered why your police force somehow didn't pursue this at the time, DS Rogers?'

Rogers shook her head. Cam could see the betrayal writ large. Not only was her own force hiding evidence, according to Chalmers, it had been deliberately avoiding solving the entire case. 'You corrupt bastard,' she said, shaking her head.

'Yes, he's a good lad, Chief Hilton, isn't he.'

Jess's eyes darted this way and that, chasing threads in her head. Abruptly, it seemed, she found two that matched, and looked up at Travis. She said two words with a quivering bottom lip. 'The … heron man.'

Cam had no idea what she meant, but she looked so pained as she spoke, he thought he could have burst. She looked at her father – or the man she had thought for so long was her dad. More threads were unspooling, giant reels of memory unravelling behind her eyes.

Tabernacle cracked. Cam saw he was crying, blubbering and drunk. 'I'm so sorry, Jess,' he said.

Jess suddenly couldn't seem to even look at her surrogate dad. Cam could almost feel the pain radiating from him as she turned away.

'You can't seriously be thinking about taking us all out there and offing us,' Cam said to Travis. *Keep their eyes on me*, he thought, as he glanced now at Chalmers. 'We've got police with us. You've got a gun for Christ's sake.'

Travis smirked. 'Police don't speak too loud when they're underwater – just like everybody else.'

'People will notice.'

'They'll only notice if they can see it. And where we're going, there's just the water and the bog and a place we can have some serious fun.'

Rogers interjected, straightening and stepping forward. 'I'm placing you under arrest for the murder of Freddie, Maud and Tommy Brindley. You do not have to say anything. But it may harm your defence if you do not mention when questioned something that you later rely on in court.'

Travis laughed as heartily as a man with no heart could. 'Have you finished?' he asked with a toothsome, canine grin.

Cam stepped forward. 'So, negotiation. You guys are businessmen, right? How do we solve this situation in a way that doesn't result in us lot being stuffed in a marsh somewhere?'

'Nothing is going to stop you from meeting that outcome,' said Travis.

Cam did his best to stay cool.

'All right. What can we do so that these innocent people can get out of here and try to put their lives back together?' Cam turned slightly to Chalmers. 'Don't you think Jess especially has been through enough?'

Chalmers walked past Cam, the gun hanging by his side, and sat on the long bench which lined the dance floor. He put a brogue upon his knee and smoothed a crease in his trouser leg. 'We're all here, so we can see this over for good. I'm not going to rest until I see the four of you silenced.'

The calm pragmatism stunned Cam. How four lives were just a nuisance factor in a business decision. It seemed to pop a valve in his chest.

He marched across to the government weasel and he already had a hand on his throat when he was rugby tack-led from behind by Danny. Cam fell hard onto the parquet, and as he pulled himself around to address the threat, he saw Danny grab that monstrous blade from his father.

'Wait!' shouted Travis. 'Wait till we're away from the village. You never know who's watching.' The old man stooped to look out of the windows suspiciously. Danny pushed Cam up onto the bench with the knife tight to his throat and scooted him up next to Chalmers.

'If you even look funny at any one of us,' he said to Cam, 'Hannah here gets gutted in front of you.'

Cam's forearms boiled as unseen forces ripped at them, his fear and panic finding new ways to torment him – but he had to beat this. For Jess. For all of them.

He looked at Danny and saw how on edge he was too. How eager to please. Cam had seen suggestions of this in the altercation at Sirens. Danny had such reverence for his father but didn't really know how to place it. It was something Cam could use. That, and something else he'd remembered.

'You don't think you can take me, do you?' Cam said, the knife still at his throat.

He tried to project that ice-cool confidence again – something that Danny was struggling with. He grimaced at the provocation. It was a spark that Cam could provoke into a fire. 'Put the knife down and let's dance. Or do you need Dad? I noticed the other two aren't here. Come on, where is all that machismo you've been aiming my way?'

Cam knew he was toying with his mortality while Danny had the blade at his throat – but if the blade was by his neck, it wasn't near Jess.

'Just wait till we get to open water,' said Danny. 'You'll find out all about me then.'

Cam put a pin in it for now, and let his taunts ferment in Danny's head while they got to where they were going.

A few more turns in the river passed by, in a strange, silent, floating stand-off – before they turned off the main river into a longer dyke that Cam knew took them to South Walsham Broad. It was another larger body of water that adorned the river system, but only a fraction of the size of Hickling.

He knew the geography of the area inside. He had studied it for hours when looking for the car. There were miles of marshland that surrounded the broad, particularly on the side they were passing through.

Cam had ruled the area out as a potential resting place of the Brindleys' Jaguar because it didn't have any roadways, contemporary or historical, which lead into the marshes. It was, however, perfect for the fulfilment of Travis's promises. A body could get lost in there, no problem.

Dread pooled: the closer they got to those marshes, the less time they had. But Cam knew he was holding an ace. He didn't know when to play it, or whether it would make any difference at this stage, but it was worth a shot.

He took inventory of everybody's positions, reasoning that there had to be at least one driver upstairs piloting the *Southern Comfort*, and perhaps another deckhand because, after all, it was a big damn boat. Whether these were the owners or not, he couldn't guess.

That meant eight, maybe nine people – only four of whom were definitely on the side of good.

He thought of situational survival chances. Not great odds when the enemy had the only two weapons.

Outside the windows, the darkness pressed in with suffocating intent. When Cam felt them turn again, this tallied with his assumptions. They had slipped off the dyke into the tributaries.

They were driving deep into the marshes.

'Quicker, quicker, hurry up,' Travis shouted, banging the knife against the ceiling, aiming his fury at the driver. He wouldn't stop looking at Cam like he wanted to skin him.

He shoved Jess next to Cam, her father on the other side next to Rogers, and the condemned four sat next to each other as they meandered towards fatality.

Cam turn to Jess and tentatively nudged his shoulder against hers.

'I'm so sorry about everything, but we're not done yet,' he said.

'I'm not really sure what's happening, I just want it to be over,' she said, and Cam could see from the hair falling over her face that she hadn't looked up. That she was trying so hard to be strong, but for something she didn't understand fully yet. She did, however, reach for his hand and rested her own on top of his for a second. 'I'm the Brindley girl, aren't I?' she whispered.

Cam didn't know how to answer. 'It … looks that way.'

'I think … I must have always known.' She still didn't look up. The turmoil, all-compassing, was etched into her expression.

Cam felt anger and regret come at him in droves, and again he told her. 'We are not done yet.'

Travis looked out the side windows, through which there was only black. He looked at his son, who nodded and stood.

'All four of you. On your knees,' Danny said. The point of the knife was aimed at the middle of the dance floor – which, after the tango of the last few days, looked like a fitting scene for an execution.

48

Cam dropped off the bench seat to his knees first, but held out an arm to prompt Jess and Tabernacle to hold fast.

'Have me,' he said. 'All this isn't necessary. It was me that caused all this, it was me that brought it all out. These people behind me just made the best of what happened to them at the time.'

Travis stepped forward, taking the knife from his son. He was smiling. 'No, no, no – if anything, you're last, and you have to take the punishment of watching them all die because you pulled them into it. You took the loose end and pulled it till the whole bloody jumper fell apart.'

He stepped to Tabernacle and grabbed the man by the hair. Tilted his head back so his whole neck was presented.

Cam looked at Chalmers, but the politician simply raised the gun and cut him off with a smirk. 'Don't look at me,' he said. 'As I'm sure you've guessed, there aren't many qualms around here about hands getting dirty.'

Cam sighed, looked at the floor where his fate was about to be dealt – and played his very last hand. 'You're still missing some pictures, aren't you?'

'You what?' Travis released Tabernacle's hair.

'Ignore him, Dad,' said Danny.

'Photographs,' said Cam. He looked at Jess. He saw a realisation, cold and bracing as an icy wind, sweep through her. Cam wished he could sit down with her and guide her carefully through what he knew – but that was impossible. He had to go with it. He looked back at Travis. 'Would it help if I could tell you where those photographs are? The real photos you're after, I mean.'

Travis stepped back in indecision and turned to look at Chalmers. Chalmers' bottom jaw floated loose, surprise cast across him.

'I'll do you a trade,' Cam said, putting his hands up in submission. 'Us four, for the photographs. You take the photographs and you turn us loose. If you don't, they'll be in the evening news, in full technicolour, before you've even got back to civilisation.'

Cam was bluffing, of course – the photographs were in his jacket pocket right then and there.

'No more bullshit,' said Travis. 'If you've seen those photographs, tell me what's in them.'

'Not with Jess present,' Cam replied. The battle with his composure was seesawing, but he was finding new reserves of strength from his sheer conviction.

The room went quiet as the stand-off bedded in, but Chalmers piped up. 'He's seen them all right.'

'Where did you get them?' asked Travis.

'Again,' Cam replied. 'Not with Jess present.'

Travis moved forward. 'He's a noble one, I'll give him that.' He grabbed Jess by the hair now and brought the knife up to her neck – but the little girl that was lost that night, and the strong woman she'd become, collided in the present.

'You killed my mother,' Jess said darkly. She swung towards him and spat a thick gob of phlegm onto the

318

bloody plaster across Travis's nose. He leaned back to hit her, and Cam broke cover with words.

'This afternoon, I found the photos at Hickling Broad.'

He didn't quite know what to say by way of follow-up. The horror of what he'd seen, and how he found it, was still almost too much to process.

Because in that wooden box, on top of a small windmill, was a huddled boy. Decomposing, skeletal, in a blue sports jacket. Cam's mind drifted with fathomless solemnity as he remembered the sight. It was the same jacket the boy had been wearing in that final photograph taken on the mayor's steps. And in that photograph, he was looking back up the steps, at who Cam was now convinced was Tyrone Travis.

Tommy, that wonderful, brave little boy, had never intended to leave his sister. He'd gone up high into the tower to look for help. Whether he'd found it was empty and climbed in for a look, or he'd been trying to hide from his bastard pursuers, it didn't matter. Tommy hadn't meant to end up stuck in there, but stuck he was.

The other side of the small entrance to the tower had been scratched to ribbons, caked in brown streaks. Blood.

And in the hands resting on his lap, clutched by those small, exposed finger bones, was a packet of photographs.

'Her brother had them,' was all he could manage to say. Tommy Brindley, found at last.

'Her brother is alive?' asked Travis, the knife drifting low in amazement.

Cam ignored him and looked at Jess. He shook his head with regret. 'I'm so sorry, Jess,' he said. 'But no. Your brother is not alive. But I have found him.'

Jess howled, the most awful connections being made in real time. It came from the depths of her stomach with a rage few would ever encounter. All those years hiding from torment, those years and a life she had pushed aside using trauma to forget … only for so many painful fragments to come back now.

She jumped to her feet and threw herself at Travis. 'Bastards!' she screamed. The old man was caught off guard and fell backwards – only to be caught by his son.

That was all the invitation Cam needed. The gun in the room be damned.

Jess Tabernacle, Hannah Brindley – she had been through enough.

He jumped to his feet and charged at Danny and Travis, tackling them both across the middle. They fell back, clattering to the dance floor, as Tabernacle and Rogers rose to take on Chalmers.

Cam lunged onto the floor to find the knife. All he found was Danny, and they grappled on the floor – giving Travis the chance to crawl out of the back door and onto the rear deck. Cam tried to reach for his trouser leg as he went, but Danny's fist caught him in the throat. He felt his windpipe crush and crumple, and he coughed and spluttered. He couldn't get enough air into his lungs, but wouldn't stop fighting with whatever breath he had left.

Opaquely, through ragged breaths, he heard the shouting behind him as Chalmers tried to keep his friends – *friends* – back with the gun. Cam spluttered again when Danny grabbed his throat and squeezed it. Cam was sure that if he survived this, he might never be able to speak again. Danny was choking him from behind, and Cam was blacking out. In his failing vision, he could just make out the sight of Chalmers thumping Johnjo on the side of the head with the gun, in a good old-fashioned pistol-whip.

He tried something new, based on a hunch – the guess that Danny had followed his father's wishes blindly through parental loyalty, without understanding the bigger picture. 'Danny … the pictures … do you want to see them?'

He felt the grip on his windpipe loosen fractionally. *Yes, Danny did.*

'I've got them, Danny. They're on me.'

'Where?' the gangster's son said.

'Jacket pocket.'

'Get them.'

Cam reached up and into his pocket and pulled out the pictures.

'Don't look at those!' came another voice.

Cam looked opposite and saw that Chalmers was standing with his legs wide, the gun pointed at the staggering Tabernacle, Rogers and Jess – but his attention was all on Danny, Cam and the pictures.

'Pull them out,' Danny said in Cam's ear. 'Show me.'

'I'm sorry, Jess,' Cam said as he opened the flap. 'Don't look, please don't look.'

He pulled out the wad of photos, angled them over his shoulder and fanned through them quickly.

'Don't you do it!' shouted Chalmers, but nobody listened, even though the gun was bouncing between targets.

'Rogers…' Cam said, his voice gravelled, appealing for the attention of the person who, legally, needed to know this the most. 'This is why the Brindleys had to die. These pictures couldn't get out.'

Cam saw the images in his periphery as he held them out for Danny to see – and with every loosening second of pressure on his neck, Cam could tell they were hitting home. He didn't really know how Danny would feel seeing those images – his gangster father and a corrupt politician having sex with a woman who'd gone missing forty years ago, all captured in the unforgiving glare of a camera flash.

But he'd seen the way Danny doted on his father, the reverence in the way he reached for him. And when he was rugby tackled by Danny at the strip club earlier, he knew the bruiser felt the same way towards his mother – because, as Danny made contact with Cam's midriff, Cam had seen the tattoo around his neck, and the word that was inscribed between the flapping wings.

Madre.

Mother.

With a dart of his hand, Cam spun one of the pictures to Rogers. 'This is why the Brindleys had to disappear. This – *this* – is what they were after.'

Paralysis seemed to grip the room. The game had been changed for so many in just a second, and it appeared that new loyalties and new boundaries had to be established. Cam felt Danny's own confusion through his neck, as the grip around him, once so tight, loosened.

'Danny,' Cam whispered. 'You were born when this happened, weren't you? Where does your own mother fit into this?'

Danny breathed into Cam's ear, and Cam could feel the confusion and rage laced within every word. 'Don't you dare mention my mother,' he said.

Cam didn't think he needed to say anything else; the point was already driven home. The rear door of the cabin opened, and a gust of cold breeze wafted in it.

'Danny, it's time to go,' said Travis, and everyone spun to look at him. He was standing in the doorway holding a bottle of spirit with a rag in the top, and in his other hand, a Bic lighter. 'What do you know, these naughty people stole this boat, they crashed it and it set on fire, and they all paid the price. Missing coppers, nuisance divers, long lost girls – oh, photographs too it seems – the whole lot went up in smoke.'

'You always were good in a pinch,' Chalmers said to Travis with a smile as he walked across the room to join him. The barrel of his pistol alternated between different people as he crossed.

'Don't get cocky, dickhead,' Travis sneered. 'If you hadn't invested that money you borrowed off me in that idiot's schemes, none of this would have been necessary.'

Tabernacle, Jess and Rogers could only watch Travis move to allow Chalmers through to the rear deck – but Danny stood furious and solid.

'Son, come on,' said Travis.

Danny looked at the photograph in his hand, and let Cam go, allowing him to stagger forward onto his haunches and breathe unrestricted for the first time in too long. It felt like every vein in his head was engorged and writhing; a side effect that Cam couldn't distinguish if it was thanks to the lack of oxygen or the lack of his meds.

Danny held the photograph, staring at the picture of his father and the MP at either end of that beautiful woman, and sat down on the bench seat. Seething.

Cam took the opportunity as if it was only one he'd ever get – and launched a punch at Danny, catching him cold on the jaw, sending him spinning.

'Sentimental prick,' bellowed Travis – before flipping the lighter, igniting the Molotov cocktail with a bright blue gush of fire. In the same motion, he flung it under-arm at the bar area. It immediately smashed with flaming spirit exploding in all directions, swallowing the optics and pumps. Other glasses smashed in the impact and burning liquid raced across the entire bar, before plunging off onto the dance floor.

The bottom deck of the *Southern Comfort* was on fire.

Cam's senses felt similarly aflame – he wanted nothing more than to dive in the water and hide beneath its cool surface – but instead he ran back to pull the Tabernacles away from the blaze, the heat of which was instantaneous.

'Go after them, you bloody idiot!' shouted Rogers, as she ran to help Jess drag the stumbling Johnjo. 'I'll get them out!'

Cam looked at the three of them, and his eyes met with Jess's. She was unbowed, whatever else was going on in there, and she nodded him on.

He turned and ran towards the rear, just in time to see Danny clambering out of one of the cabin's side windows, hauling himself into the darkness.

Cam emerged on the rear deck, into the fresh, biting marsh air. Another engine started, a smaller one that buzzed at a higher frequency than the boats main engine, and it started to rev.

'Cast us off,' Chalmers shouted from somewhere. Cam looked over the side behind the unused paddle, to find a dinghy roped to the larger cruiser.

The getaway vehicle. This had been the plan all along – to leave the *Southern Comfort* burned to a crisp deep in the marshes, where the emergency services couldn't reach it in time. But when they did, they'd find the charred bodies of a handful of unidentifiable joy riders – if they found anything at all. They would just be another secret lost to the marsh, and the water of the Norfolk Broads.

Below, in the dinghy, were Travis and Chalmers, at the engine with his pistol. He cracked off a potshot at Cam, but it sailed harmless and wild over his head into the black sky. Travis reached for the mooring rope and untethered the dinghy.

The engine revved, the water at the rear of the dinghy turned white, and in a heartbeat and a surge of blistering clarity, Cam threw himself over the side at the small boat.

49

Rogers emerged from the cabin of the *Southern Comfort*, just in time to see Cam's legs disappearing over the side and into the black. She ran to the railing and looked down – just as a gunshot cracked the night in half. She'd been lucky. It was a wild shot but it couldn't have been far away. Nevertheless, she remembered what she'd seen. Cam landing in the middle of a small dinghy, in between Travis and Chalmers. There was shouting and the rev of an outboard being kicked into full throttle. She hunkered down in case any more shots were fired, and glanced back at the cabin.

Smoke was billowing fast, even though they were still moving.

She paused.

We're still moving.

The pilot was still up there.

Next to the cabin door was the stairs up to the top deck.

'Find a fire extinguisher!' she shouted to Jess, as the recently revealed Hannah Brindley guided Johnjo onto a double seat overlooking the rear paddles.

Jess simply nodded back. Rogers took the rear steps two at a time.

I couldn't get the arrest down there, she thought. *I'll be damned if I'm missing one up here.*

Cam landed in the boat with a painful thunk, right across the middle bench. His ribs took most of the impact, but there was no time to think because, just as the pain registered and flooded across his torso like a spilt drink, the engine was jacked into its highest gear, the throttle twisted to its noisiest extremity. With the noise came the unbalancing surge in speed, and he fell back into the bottom of the boat.

'Jesus, shoot him!' shouted Travis, reminding Cam, as if he needed it, of the imminent danger of Chalmers' gun – although Cam thought the political behemoth was in fact uncomfortable with shooting. When Chalmers had pulled a shot in his direction moments before, his aim had been so bad, that it might well have been on purpose.

The gun, however, cold and autonomous, would have no such compunction – and Cam always respected their power. He reached for Chalmers' leg, which he'd crashed against when the acceleration threw him, and went for another of his favoured ankle twists – but Chalmers clubbed him with the butt of the pistol. His ear rang like a church bell crashing down the spire itself as more blows rained down. He loosened his grip to allow his elbow to move left, and protect his ear, and Chalmers wriggled free.

'Shoot him!' screamed Travis again – but the struggle had obviously affected Chalmers' control of the dinghy, as it bumped alongside the flaming flank of the Mississippi steamboat.

Cam saw the gun come down above him, not in a strike this time, but with more control as its open barrel swung towards him – so he lunged for the tiller again, lurching the dinghy sideways and into the flank of the larger burning boat once more. It caused the two men standing to wobble, but not Cam, on his knees. At the lowest centre of gravity, he was quicker to adjust, and rose to grab Chalmers' wrist. They were locked in a battle over the control of the pistol.

Travis started to walk towards them, holding an oar over his head. 'Jesus, just shoot the bastard!' he shouted, swinging the oar at Cam.

Cam half-caught the oar and hit the tiller again, this time the other way, and the momentum of the swinging oar and the turning boat caught the old man off guard. He tumbled head first into the open water and his entire body slipped beneath the black surface.

The top deck was dim and eerily quiet, and Rogers mused that you'd be forgiven for thinking there was no fire below them at all. The cabin space was enclosed by all-weather covering, with plastic bench seats bolted in rows right the way to the front – where the helm sat in its own wooden cuddy. At the wheel, was a man in a black jacket, with a bottle of wine at his elbow. There was no glass in sight, and there was simply a plastic straw popped in the neck. It gave Rogers the impression the man was not pleased to be here, and was drinking his way through the occasion.

She stayed low, and slunk between the rows, her eyes never leaving the back of the pilot's head. He seemed steadfastly oblivious to what was going on downstairs. Rogers caught a tinny sound over the engine throb, something high-pitched.

Music. He had tunes on in there.

She readied her warrant card, in her right hand, has she approached the cabin door, reaching with her left.

Words hadn't worked last time. This time, she'd make sure the threat was nullified before she attempted the arrest.

She hadn't often had to engage in roughhousing as a cop, but she had no problem getting her hands dirty when she was a police constable earning her stripes in nineties Norwich. It had been a while, however.

Now or never.

For Tommy, she thought, and threw open the door.

The change in direction made Cam and Chalmers separate, with the former staggering back towards the middle of the boat, before tripping on that damn middle bench seat again. He landed painfully on his backside as he looked up at Chalmers, who smiled once again.

'This is all coming up rather well. One less loose end to worry about,' he said, as he drew the gun up to Cam's eyes. Cam waited for the gunshot to sound – but it didn't. Instead, Chalmers' eyes widened at what was ahead – where the boat was going.

The boat abruptly came to a stop as they hit something. It was Chalmers' turns to fall forward, as Cam slid towards the nose. He sat up and looked around, and in the flickering glow of the blazing steamboat, saw that they had driven into a floating reed bed – essentially a chunk of marsh, a living ecology all of its own, that had broken off and was floating randomly through the bog.

And now, they were stuck in it.

The engine shorted out with the exertion of going nowhere, and the only sound was the crackle and billow of the lower half of the *Southern Comfort* being swallowed by flames.

Cam prayed that his friends had got off that boat.

He lunged across to where Chalmers had fallen, his long peacoat now covered in the debris that had accumulated on the boat's floor, and straddled the man's back.

'Where's the gun, Chalmers?' he shouted, as Chalmers bucked beneath him. It appeared over the man's right shoulder, and fire spat from the barrel with a deafening blast. Cam had to recoil, and as he did, he felt a wet hand on his neck.

'Come here, you bastard,' a grizzled voice croaked, and Cam swung his head to see Travis, soaked and furious, pulling himself up over the back of the boat – the engine in one hand, and Cam's collar in the other.

Cam sailed backwards and was practically sucked into the black water. Most people would have been panicked at the abrupt plunge into the icy drink, but Cam felt the cool grip of the water as a welcome pressure across every inch of his skin. He felt Travis's arms around him, squeezing him, pushing him deeper, but he didn't fight it.

He let the cold quiet work its way into him, restoring him in the way it always had, and waited a moment.

This was Cam's world, where he felt at his most safe, his most normal, his strongest. This was his turf.

As soon as Travis released his grip so he could get air himself, Cam surged upwards to meet him at the surface. They both burst into the air at the same time, Travis with a gasp for breath, and Cam with a swinging fist into Travis's gaping mouth. He felt jagged teeth on his knuckles as they cracked under the speed and force of his fist.

Aware he needed to get back to Chalmers, who still had the gun, he grabbed the side of the dinghy, and threw his arms up and over, hauling himself into the small vessel. He was quickly aboard again and saw Chalmers pulling himself up near the bow – but Travis's rough, soaking hands grabbed Cam again from behind, yanking him back towards the water.

Cam fought for balance, and reached for the only thing he could – the engine's tiller and its ignition switch. He hit it, and as the engine roared to life, the water around the back of the boat frothed immediately – and with it came a scream so raw with pain, it hurt the very soul.

Travis let go of Cam, and Cam turned to see the old man straddling the engine from behind like he was trying to ride it. The engine juddered as its propellor tore through Travis, and the water around him foamed fuchsia. The old man fell back into a soup of his own blended viscera, his face looking at the heavens, his arms outstretched as if he acknowledged his deeds had finally come to challenge him, and would embrace the accumulated punishment with open arms.

Cam's horror at the sight was short-lived when the hammer of the gun clicked behind his head.

As Rogers pulled open the cabin door, the sweet-stale odour of wine breath escaped the small space, alongside the crashing chorus of Tina Turner's 'We Don't Need Another Hero (Thunderdome)'. She pushed through, and launched into the pilot. He fell forward, his flailing arms knocking the wine bottle, spilling claret all over the console as if the man had suffered an arterial wound.

She abruptly grabbed his right arm, and shoved it so far up his back he could have been puppeteering himself. He yelped.

'Stop the boat,' she said into his ear.

'Yes, yes!' he said, as he used his other arm to pull back on the throttle.

'Tina Turner, really?'

'They told me to stay up here, put some music on and drive us out into the marshes. They told me not to leave this cabin until they came to tell me otherwise. The old man had a big knife, said he'd use it on my family!'

'Are you the normal pilot?'

'Yes!'

Sensing minimal threat from the half-cut man, she span him round. 'Bloody hell, what is that? Smells like toilet cleaner.'

'It's the onboard merlot.'

'Which one's the anchor?'

He pointed shakily to a button which had a large sticker of an anchor on it. Rogers pressed it, and immediately heard heavy clunking somewhere below.

'Are you going to be a good boy?' she asked sternly.

'Yes,' the man said pleadingly.

'I don't need to cuff you?'

'No!'

'Then follow me. Your boat's on fire by the way.'

'What?'

Rogers turned and guided the increasingly shell-shocked man back across the top deck to the rear.

'Now that really is one less loose end to worry about,' Chalmers said. 'And you've finally wiped my debts with it.'

Cam, too tired and stunned to care much anymore, put his hands up and turned to face the politico. 'You borrowed money off him, didn't you? And you invested that money with Freddie Brindley. He lost everything and you found yourself tied to a loan shark.'

'Not the best decision I've ever made, granted. And he's got such a… *direct* way of going about things.'

332

Cam shook his head. 'Aren't you tired, Chalmers?' he said. 'Aren't you just completely exhausted with all this running?'

'If you want a career in politics, my boy, running is the name of the game.'

'I know why you want them buried, Chalmers. I know...' Cam replied. 'It would kill it before it started wouldn't it?'

Chalmers' bravado finally seemed to suffer a blow. 'How do you...'

'You're not the only one who knows people's backstories.'

Chalmers took a second before grimacing. 'You know fuck all, Killick.' His eyes drifted to the distance, and the flaming steamboat. It was really going up now, with pieces of trim tumbling to the water, and the flames reaching up into the second deck and roof. It wouldn't be long before the whole thing was gone.

'What if I told you those photographs are copies,' Cam said. 'And will be on the front page nationally, whatever you do next?'

Chalmers just smirked. 'I'd tell you you're a fool to think I couldn't get back to civilisation and stop it. I've got every newspaper editor on speed dial.'

The two men faced each other, the burning pyre of the huge vessel, crackling and crumbling in the background.

'But someone would see it. Someone would notice and remember the face. Especially now you're so close to becoming a duke.'

'How...'

'What does a man with seemingly endless power want? Turns out it's even more power.'

Cam set his jaw and said nothing. Gupta and Ferris had come up with the goods. They'd found the current Duke of Norfolk was deep into his nineties, and now on end-of-life care, and connected the dots as to what would come next. The problem was, this duke sadly had no living heirs, which meant the title would become extinct. However, the Duke of Norfolk was no ordinary dukedom. The King would most likely raise someone else to the title, to carry on the tradition, because this was the premier dukedom, elevating the holder to huge importance, not just in its close links to the royal family, but in a wider historical sense. The Duke of Norfolk assumed the role of Earl Marshall, and would organise state funerals, coronations and the like. It was as close as you could get to becoming part of the royal family, without being born into it.

Cam imagined Chalmers would love all that acclaim, but not as much as the other bonus that came with the title; almost fifty thousand acres of land – and all the rental income to go with it. The dukedom, in short, offered instant, eye-watering riches. And who was in line for the position?

Norfolk's longest serving member of the House of Lords, and all-round political stalwart, Lord Chalmers.

In an era of royal scrutiny, and a government vowing overhaul of the peerages process, those photos would ruin him before he'd even been anointed.

'I'd get away with it,' Chalmers said. 'I always do. A previous PM was caught arranging the beating of a journalist, for Christ's sake. A living prince managed to get himself involved in a worldwide sex-trafficking ring. A little sexscapade is nothing.' But the look in Chalmers' eyes suggested he didn't quite believe his own words.

The contempt Cam felt for this man was almost overwhelming. The gun was inches from his face, yet, somehow, he felt no fear. He'd come this far, and frankly, looking at

Chalmers right now, he was convinced that he and the bullet in that gun would have no future together.

'You've never pulled the trigger, have you?' said Cam, looking steadily back down the barrel at Chalmers. 'Not with intent.'

Chalmers didn't answer.

'You've always had someone do it for you, haven't you?' Chalmers stopped breathing, and Cam knew he had him. He wanted him to fire. He wanted him to commit.

'You've not got it in you.' But Cam saw the decision had been made and the trigger was going to be pulled. All this latency, however, and Chalmers' obvious agonising over firing, gave Cam the slightest warning.

He jabbed his head to the right, as the gun went off in his left ear.

He wouldn't hear out of it for a while, but it was better than a bullet being stuck in the grey matter next to it.

As Cam expected, the shock of the pistol's recoil took Chalmers by surprise, and his hand bucked aimlessly skyward as the shot echoed off into the wilderness.

Cam grabbed the gun, twisted it out of the stunned politician's hand and pointed it at him. Chalmers looked like a rat stuck in the corner while the terrier waited for it to move.

'You'll confess to everything when I take you in,' Cam said.

'No one would believe you,' said the politician, even as his hands shot up. 'All the evidence of any of this is stuck on that boat.'

Cam glanced back at the burning *Southern Comfort* and caught sight of his friends, on the rear deck. They were tackling the cabin blaze with fire extinguishers. He wanted to get to them. *Fast.*

'There's always this,' Cam said, pulling a solitary photograph from his sock. He held it up in the flickering light
for Chalmers to see – and for Chalmers to fully realise
that, finally, the game was up.

The photo showed Chalmers engaged in intercourse
with Maud Brindley on the night she died – along with
Travis, a well-known loan shark. And in Maud Brindley's
eyes, were tears.

The Lord looked at the picture, hoping to conjure one
last way out. But even he, the slipperiest of politicos who
had made a career out of greasing hands, couldn't find a
way out. He looked at the picture and sighed.

Cam had kept it separate from the rest of the pack, just
in case, as an insurance policy, wrapped around his lower
calf and held in place by the sock elastic. An ace pulled
secretly from the main deck. The image was probably the
most damning picture of the lot, and Cam didn't even
want to think about it. Somehow however, the contorted
shapes of the bodies in those photographs still managed
to make the sleazy politician smile. 'It was a hell of a run,'
said Chalmers.

'Freddie Brindley took the photographs, the stupid,
stupid man. He thought bringing his children to the
party would stop us from having our way with his lovely
wife – the interest charged on him fucking up so grandly.
Then he photographed the bloody thing. Attempted to
blackmail us. You can imagine, pictures floating about
of a serving government official having sex with someone that wasn't his wife – in a threesome with a known
criminal, no less – were potentially very bad for business. We did everything we could to get our hands on
those pictures. *Everything.* Of course … it went a bit far.
Then it became pictures of an MP having sex with a

missing woman, and … well, you can imagine how it would look.'

'Even though it was the truth, no matter how it looked.'

Chalmers waved his hand dismissively. 'Whatever. Turns out, Brindley's boy had them all along.'

'And he died holding all your secrets.'

'Well, yes. I haven't seen those pictures in forty years. Any chance you could let me have that one, as a little going away present?' Chalmers smiled lecherously.

'It was all just to protect your reputation then. So you could hold on to power. You didn't mind whose lives you wrecked as long as you could keep yours. If those kids ever came back and identified you, and if those pictures were ever found, you knew your career would be over in disgrace. You make me sick,' Cam said, and he smashed the butt of the gun into the side of Chalmers' head.

Cam took the tiller and gunned it back to the boat, but the engine juddered and made heavy weather of the short trip. The fire was now consuming the top deck, but he could see his friends were still at the back. Rogers was holding the rest of the photographs and waved them in his direction. She'd got the whole lot off Danny. That was something.

As Cam pulled alongside them. 'Are you all OK?' he called to the three. No, four. There was a man in a white shirt and life vest he didn't recognise, who was staring at the flames with his hands on his head. The pilot, maybe.

Cam took them all in, but his heart kept reaching for Jess. He looked at her. She looked strong yet wounded, still alive, and ready to get the hell out of there. She had her left hand in her surrogate father's right.

'We're hanging in there,' she said.

337

Cam smiled. 'Everybody on.'

Hurriedly, the four lowered themselves into the boat. As Rogers passed him, she put a hand on his shoulder. 'You are a wonder, Cam Killick,' she said. He could tell she meant it. 'Can you take me to poor old Tommy in the morning?'

Cam gave her the gun and a sad smile. 'Yes…' he said. 'When Jess is sorted. This is a lot for her to take in at this point.'

'Of course. We'll go higher than Hilton on this. This is bigger than him, and we can prove it all.'

He smiled at Rogers and nodded. He reached to give her a hug, but she snapped at him:

'Even after escaping a fiery death, I'm not hugging you, Killick.'

He stepped back, revved the engine hard, which only caused it to gargle and churn, before it gave up with a deep clunk. He looked over the back of the engine, down at the propellor. It was in a bad way, considering what had been fed through it just moments earlier, and he didn't want to spend too much time investigating.

'No bother,' he said, turning back. 'Who's up for rowing?'

Before his last word had even rung out, a high-pitched whining could be heard over the billow of the flames from the boat behind them. It was coming from back towards the entrance to the marshes and the broads beyond.

Cam squinted, until he started to see two bright orange shapes, coming towards them. They were on the water. The drone got louder, as the shapes got closer.

Cam smiled, and shook his head in disbelief.

It was another dinghy, heading towards them, emblazoned with the words 'Horning Sailing Club'. And kneeling in the vessel, clad in two of the most oversized lifejackets he'd ever seen, were Gupta and Ferris.

Ferris was filming everything with her phone, while Gupta steered closer. 'We arrived at the pub just as the boat was leaving. Saw you through the windows. We followed you as best we could but this thing's quite a bit slower!' Gupta shouted then pointed at the flames. 'That's quite the rescue beacon you've got!' She pulled alongside them. Ferris kept looking from the fire to the sky overhead.

'It wasn't aliens, Ferris,' Cam shouted.

'That's what you think,' she replied.

Tabernacle and Gupta roped the boats together, and Cam took one last look at the *Southern Comfort*, as it stood over the reeds, blazing uncontrollably, another sacrifice to the Broadland waters.

Cam felt a hand in his own and turned to see Jess. She looked on the cusp of tears, but she managed to smile.

He didn't know what to say, as she rested her head on his shoulder. 'We'll get you right,' he managed. He looked across at Johnjo Tabernacle, whose own eyes were streaming.

'It's the smoke,' he said, pulling a laugh from Cam.

Jess's hand squeezed his – and it gave him more strength than any tablet or trip underwater ever had.

50

The plane ride was horrendous.

Everything Cam hated about enclosed spaces and human beings mashed together in planes. He had to use breathing exercises the whole time, even though the flight was relatively short, and he'd been sensible with his meds earlier that day to give him the best chance of making the journey without going into full meltdown. His dose was reduced, and while some days were better than others, he was making progress.

The drive was better, into the countryside and mountains of the Pyrenees, the vineyard country of southern France. Quiet, green and blissful, it was a world away from the cut and thrust of the endless police interviews he'd endured, although they were made easier by the fact that Rogers had backed him to the hilt in every single one of them. The police couldn't deny Chalmers' confessions, including those about paying high-ranking officers to keep the Brindley matter quiet, and senior heads on the force were rolling. Nevertheless, Rogers extolled Cam's heroism in the face of disaster and fought with a granite backbone for the justice of the children. Jess had been interviewed too, and it had depleted both of them. She was remembering more and more, and he'd supported her throughout – but it had been just so damn *painful*. When it was all over, he was happy just to leave, and never wanted to talk about the situation, the events of that car ever again.

He did, however, have one last thing to take care of.

Travis and Chalmers had been obsessed with loose ends, and Cam had been left with one that was impossible to ignore. It came to him when he met Tabernacle, after Rogers had originally told him to leave the case alone. Belvedere, was the name. It had taunted him, right from the very beginning, right from when he first discovered the resting place of the Brindley Jaguar.

Belvedere.

The name of the company that owned that stretch of land on Hickling Broad.

Cam had kept looking, even though the car had been found. He researched Belvedere. It had led him to Belvedere Inc. in France, with a registered office address in Corsavy. And that was how he found himself walking up the steps to a countryside chateau peppered with flourishing vines and stone balustrades. This was where the trail ended. From here, there was nowhere else to go.

He rang the front doorbell, as the grey skies pulled to murk. Rain began to fall. And as soon as the door was answered, he knew he was in the right place.

Belvedere.

'Yes?' said the man who opened the door.

'Good evening,' Cam said. 'I'm sorry to disturb you like this, but may I come in?'

The man, who had to be in his seventies, looked at him with tired eyes and dishevelled confusion. 'An Englishman? What are you doing all the way out here?'

'I think it would be better for you if I came inside,' Cam said, firmly. 'I've come all the way from Norfolk.'

Those eyes suddenly ignited. 'I suppose you better had.'

Cam went inside the impressive house. He was led into a living room, clad with books. There were no photographs to speak of at all; no art hung on the walls, no memories anywhere.

The man dropped himself heavily into an armchair, and looked at Cam uncertainly. Even though age had made inroads upon him, the Hollywood handsomeness was still there, amid the grey hairs and haunted expression.

He pointed to one of the other armchairs, on which Cam sat.

After a moment of silence, Cam decided there was no room for preamble, and went straight to it. 'Not so long ago, I found your green Jaguar.'

Freddie Brindley froze, his eyes blitzed wide with shock.

'I've spent the last few days with the police. Going over everything I know about Hickling Broad, Lord Chalmers and Tyrone Travis. They don't know I'm here – I've saved this part for myself. The thing I can't work out,' he said, 'is why. Why did you choose to appease both Travis and Chalmers by offering them your *wife*?'

Freddie searched for words, his jaw moving, but nothing emerged.

Cam spoke again. 'And then, why did *you* get to survive this, and your children and wife didn't?'

Opposite Cam, Freddie crumpled with resignation, as if these were questions he'd always expected to answer one day, but had never truly believed that day would come. His eyes were glazed, and his grey fringe flopped long over his brow. He pushed it impatiently aside. After a moment, he found his voice. It was angry.

'What has this got to do with you? What has any of this got to do with you?!'

'Because I know it all, Freddie. And I could tell them. I could have the gendarmes knocking on that door just like I did. All it would take is a phone call. But I don't want to. I don't think it should be my call. So I just want to know *why*.'

'Chalmers was in the hole,' he said. 'Gambling. But the world was moving on without him, and he wanted in on the big scores in the finance sector. He borrowed money from a local loan shark to fund his investments with me. And the loan shark was not happy when all that money disappeared.'

The bare pragmatism in his words stunned Cam.

'So, Chalmers chose to ruin you unless you fixed it. He said use of your wife was merely "interest" paid after a business deal had gone wrong.' Cam struggled to keep the repulsion out of his voice.

'We both agreed it,' Freddie burst out. 'They threatened the children if we didn't come up with something. I thought it might keep them happy while I fixed things.'

'And your wife hated you for it.'

'I didn't know what else to do.' Freddie couldn't even look at Cam.

'But you took pictures, didn't you?' Cam said.

'I did. I honestly thought it would get me out of everything. Get me off what I owed Chalmers, and in turn what he owed Travis. But they … didn't see it like that.'

'And the children?' Cam asked gravely.

Freddie put his head in his hands. 'They were in the car, I didn't think for one second they'd actually do anything, not to the children, but the car drifted out of sight with them in it. I couldn't tell them where the pictures were.

343

They had guns to our heads, and … Travis let the children float away.' Freddie looked white, his face sagging with detachment, like saying the words out loud at last was the most potent horror.

'And they shot Maud,' Cam said.

'Yes,' Freddie whispered. 'But how do you know?'

'I had a natter with Tyrone Travis about the very topic.'

Freddie closed his eyes as if horrified at the return of *that* name from the past. When he opened them, they were far away, as if he was reliving it all over again. 'They took me back to our home. Told me to get rid of the body and prove I didn't have the photos. I'd just watched my family die, I had no reason to keep it from them anymore. I didn't have them, no matter how much they hit me. They told me to disappear forever – and if I ever came back, they'd make sure everyone knew I killed my family.'

'And then what? They just let you go?'

'I truly wish they had killed me. But they said that leaving me alive, knowing that I was responsible for the deaths of my wife and children … well, it would be the greatest punishment of all.'

'And was it?'

Freddie looked at Cam with eyes red and bloodshot. 'I'm living in hell. Have been since that night.'

'So you bought that stretch of water and set up protection over Brindley Hall so that nobody would discover the truth. The horrible mistakes you'd made. You let your own children die, let your wife get shot, to save your own skin. Didn't you?'

Freddie glared at him. 'Say what you want – I've given myself more punishment tenfold.'

'I'll tell you what I will say – or rather what I'm sure of. This is a nice set up for a guy who lost a lot of money and ran away with nothing.'

'What are you implying?' said Freddie indignantly, but Cam could see the fear.

'Black Monday was very convenient, wasn't it?'

Freddie looked at him, and an air of desperation entered his expression.

'Nothing like a good international financial disaster to hide stealing from your clients, is there?'

Freddie didn't say anything.

Cam did. 'You didn't lose your clients' money. You stole it, and made it look like it was all part of Black Monday. All of this, every brick of this chateau is paid for by your family's blood. I hope you feel proud of yourself. I hope it was worth it.'

Freddie stammered, looked everywhere but at Cam, and eventually rested his eyes on the ground at his feet. 'It wasn't supposed to go that way. We were supposed to all be here, starting anew, away from all those bloody people.'

Cam was disgusted. He thought about all that Brindley had confirmed, and realised the obvious blanks – the children. Cam was now sure that Freddie had no idea what really happened to Hannah and Tommy.

But that wasn't his story to tell. And that led to the second reason why he was here.

January 2025

I hit the doorbell, unable to wait any longer.

I'd told Cam I'd wait for him to make the initial introductions and to make sure that he was ready to see me.

But I don't care what he thinks. He's already had enough from me. I want him to see me. I want him to see firsthand that despite what they all did, I'm still here.

I thought I'd be scared. When I first found out my dad wasn't my real father, it somehow didn't feel that new. Like on a very deep, subconscious level, the knowledge was already there.

A lot came flooding back. Loads.

I remembered that night, or at least a couple of bits of it. That dog did it, the one that was on Cam's nightstand at Hotel Wroxham. A door was thrown open deep down, and memories crawled through into the light like unexpected goblins. That dog is in my bag, right now by my side. I've not been without it since Cam gave it back to me.

I'm not nervous. I'm proud.

I'm Jess Tabernacle.

Not the girl these people let die.

I can hear movement beyond the door. Footsteps.

I should feel fear now, I know I should. But I don't.

I feel defiant.

The door swings open, and I know it's my father before I've even seen him properly. The man who abandoned us. He didn't even try to come looking for us. He just ran away, a coward.

I'm full of pity. It surprises me, because the pity is not for myself, but for him.

His face, when he sees me, fills with a pained recognition. It can't have been easy for him, living with what he did. But it was no picnic for me either.

The memories of my lost seven years are hard to make peace with. The pain of realising what my parents had done is even worse.

'Hannah,' he says, and his hand comes up. It hovers a foot from my face, an invitation to touch.

I don't take it.

'Jess,' I say, holding my position. 'It's Jess now.'

My first father smiles, and bares his teeth in doing so – but as soon as I see his canines, the smile turns into a painful grimaced sob.

Not my father any more. His grey hair is shoulder length now, his tan assured despite the time of year. His blue eyes, once so handsome, look depthless, a diamond revealed to have been false all along.

'Hannah,' he says.

'Jess,' I correct him again.

Behind him, behind the man who *should* have been my saviour, is one of the men who actually did save me. My dad Johnjo, and this man, Cam Killick. I can almost imagine my brother Tommy here beside me. Cam gives me that

347

look. The one he's been giving me since I first met him. The one that asks, *are you OK?*

I nod firmly.

'I can't believe you're alive … Jess,' Freddie says.

'Yes. Surprising what goes on behind your back when you don't give a damn,' I say. This visit is for me. Not them. This is closure for *me.*

But there's another reason.

'I came to tell you,' I say, my legs so rooted to the doorstep I feel like I can feel the earth's core through my soles, 'that while I survived, Tommy didn't.'

That causes a stony, wide-eyed silence from Freddie.

'We both got out of the car. He pulled me to safety, like a true hero. Then he told me he was going to get help. As far as we can tell, he climbed an observation tower not a hundred metres from where the car went in the water. Probably looking for help. God knows why, but he climbed into the maintenance box on the top. He died of hypothermia. If only you had looked that night, you'd have found us both. But you didn't, and he died carrying your secret with him. He protected you to the very end, and for many years after.'

'He knew?' Freddie asks. His jaw hangs open and his teeth are visible. It's a kind of horrified grimace – and I think it's directed at himself.

'He knew everything. He had the photographs.'

The photographs … the ones that got us all in so much trouble. The ones that got Tommy and my birth mother killed.

'We couldn't tell them where they were, no matter how much they asked!' Freddie shouts. 'If only he'd given them to us, none of this would have happened.'

348

I step to him. 'Don't you dare blame him for what happened. Don't you *dare*.'

He stands, chastened. The sad little man who always wanted to be the big dog, reduced to a whelp.

'I came here for something – and then I never want to hear from you again.'

'Oh, Jess,' Freddie pleaded, stepping forward again.

'Step back, Freddie, that ship sailed when you sent the rest of your family to their deaths.'

'I understand,' Freddie says, his hands floating at his sides like their connection to his brain has just been severed.

'We buried Tommy last week,' I say. 'I want to do the same for my mother.'

I hear crows cry, somewhere in the branches overhead, and I know they're not for me. It feels foreboding. It feels like my father's darkness has finally been realised.

'Now. Where is my mother's body?'

He can't ignore me. Not when I'm standing in front of him. When I know, I can bury my mother and Tommy next to each other, together. At last.

After a few silent moments, Freddie Brindley tells us where Maud is, and a lost piece of me, however strangely, falls back into place.

Epilogue

Cam took the huge tendril of knotweed and pulled it hard. The root was deeply embedded out there beneath the water, so he had to really put his back into it from the bank. He glanced down to his left, as he spread his legs apart in a lunge to get better purchase, and saw Nala, watching him with a humorous expression.

'Oh, you want a turn?' he asked her. She merely huffed in response, dismissively. Next to her was a cream ball of fluff. 'How about you?'

Cam looked at the new dog, Wicket, a Shorkie just like Nala, except his snout carried more of the Shih Tzu lineage, and he had a little underbite nestled beneath his pug nose. He remained motionless. 'Didn't think so.'

He took the strain and with two hands pulled the thick rope of weed as hard as he could. At last it broke free, and with it released a bubble of trapped gas and air up to the surface of the lake next to Brindley Hall. He pulled the mess back to the bank, end over end, and threw it on the wheelbarrow with the other grubby tentacles he had pulled out throughout the morning.

As he tucked the remaining fingers into the wheelbarrow, he glanced around the estate. It was much neater than before. The lawn had been mown back and reseeded, ready for the spring to make it green again. The vines had been stripped from the walls of Brindley Hall itself, and Jess and Johnjo had given it a brilliant white paint job. The entire foliage had been gradually beaten back, and Cam had run out of counting how many bonfires they had lit to burn through the accumulated greenery. The windows were clear and shining, and the place looked worlds away from how it had been only a few short winter months prior.

Cam would have helped, but his duty, once again, lay with the water.

'Are you calling it a day yet?' asked a voice from behind him.

He turned. Sat on the bottom step of Brindley Hall, underneath its circular-balustraded entrance, were Jess and Johnjo. They were in jeans and wellington boots, and had taken off their jackets to enjoy the midday sun. Jess looked comfortable enough – although it was only in the last two weeks that she had taken to staying here.

It was only these last three nights that Cam had stayed there, too.

'Not yet,' he shouted back. Jess smiled at him, softly but burned through with warmth.

'Be careful,' she shouted.

He smiled back. He saw how nervous she was – and Johnjo evidently saw it too, putting an arm around his daughter. Cam turned and pulled his mask over his eyes, adjusted the straps to the tank on his back, and walked back into the lake.

His was a strange, thankless task, but it had made him and Jess stronger, somehow. As if a shared resilience in the face of life's macabre tricks had fused them together.

He wiped the slime and mud off his hands onto the bare legs beneath his board shorts, his arms no longer carrying the frantic buzz of anxiety. Which was surprising because he'd been off all medication for bearing on two months.

It had been a sensible, controlled weaning, as he allowed the drugs to leave his system, bit by bit, with the support of the one person he knew he could trust above all else. He admired Jess until the ends of the earth, the way she was rebuilding herself brick by brick, and reclaiming her heritage in a way she was happy with. Further to that, she had his back and he had hers, and he couldn't think, not after all they'd been through, anything in the world would change that. And amidst that, he'd realised something.

As time went by, and opportunities and happiness flicked past in the blink of an eye, it was OK to go for them. That when good things happened, and positives emerged in your life, you were well within your right to reach for them with both hands and hold on tight.

He slipped beneath the surface into that dark, dank world once again.

Tipping forward, he began to paddle, his arms by his side in the shape of a slow and methodical torpedo. He memorised where he was headed. Where the knotweed had popped up.

The lake was much clearer now since the first time he'd dived it some months ago. He'd scraped, dredged and cleared the bottom as best he could, all part of his search.

Other people could have done this, but Cam wanted the responsibility himself. He had the experience and the expertise as much as anyone else. But above all that, he wanted to do it for Jess.

And while she and her father had been cleaning and renovating on dry land, he'd been steadily trawling through the depths nearby, pulling out piece by overgrown piece, searching.

He'd had no luck so far – but in the dark green swirls ahead, he saw a long black shape on the bottom. Right where the ripped-out knotweed had been.

The familiar charge of electricity shot through him.

Inching closer, he saw the shape more clearly, partially covered in silt and slime, the rest swiped off as the knotweed holding it in place had been removed.

It was clearly the right size.

Wrapped tightly in black bags.

A rope tied around the middle of the parcel, with the other half-tied to a rusted barbell, almost completely sunken, just two ridges of coppered metal poking out from the silt.

Maud Brindley, just as Freddie had described.

He rose to the surface and trod water, removing his mask.

'Jess,' he shouted. At the house, both she and Johnjo jumped up.

'Have you got her?' Jess shouted. Her eyes contained a strained mix of horror and hope.

'It's over, Jess,' he said. She clasped her hands in front of her face as Johnjo held her tight.

It's over, he thought, as he pulled the mask over his eyes, and went beneath the rolling surface one last time.

A Note from the Author

This book could be seen as a dark love-letter to Norfolk. Any similarities in these pages to real events and people are entirely coincidental, while so many of the places are real. Any errors are mine, and unintentional – unless something had to be eased into a different place or shape for narrative purposes. Thank you for continuing to give me so many happy memories, and inspiring me in every way possible.

Acknowledgements

First and foremost in my mind is always my wife and children. Becky, Ava, Sylvia and Robin.

Thank you for letting daddy do what he does, I love you all like you wouldn't believe. I'm the luckiest guy in the world.

My family is immeasurably important to me, and I'm grateful to them all. My parents Andy and Alex have made so much possible through sheer force of love, for which I could never thank them enough, and my siblings and my siblings-in-law all play giant roles every day in ways they might never know. Jonny, Susie, Lauren and Matt, thank you. You also gave me a team of nieces and nephews who I adore, and who make me endlessly happy. Charlotte, Abigail, Max and Harry, I'm so proud to be your uncle.

Graham and Dru, I couldn't be more grateful for the love, inspiration and support you continue to give us. Thank you always for the way you invited me into your family.

To my wider family, and everyone in it – I love you all, and thank you. They say you can't choose your family – I'm afraid I'd still have chosen you.

The question of family is a great one, because in the book world, I feel like I've expanded mine, and made all new ones.

My new Bloomsbury Raven family, I'm so happy to be working with you, and really thank my lucky stars I get to work with such glittering minds. To my editor Therese Keating, I will always be grateful – for taking a chance on me and this book, and for making it so much better in every way. I'm sure you are already sick of me saying thank you, but it's genuine. Fabrice Wilmann, Wilhelmina Asaam, thank you so much for all your efforts, the mysterious 'Ben' in marketing who came up with the title (which works so much better), Charlotte Phillips for the wonderful cover, thank you. To everyone at Bloomsbury who ever took a look at that 'cold case diver' book, thank you for everything you have done and continue to do. I feel one lucky boy.

To Siofra O'Connor and Stacia Briggs, thank you so very much for letting me use your story as an inspiration. Anyone familiar with your own story and careers will recognise immediately where I might have got the idea of the characters of Gupta and Ferris, and, while those characters are entirely fictional creations for storytelling purposes, their inclusion really is a tribute to the sheer coolness of what you do, and a thank you for the many happy hours of listening you have given me with the Norfolk Folklore Society podcast. That podcast, and the pair of you, are inspiration on tap. Thank you for letting me do this.

There's a number of people I'd like to thank for reasons only they might understand. Pamela Eccleston, the Circle of Trust, Heleen Kist, Sarah Moorhead, Danny Middleton, Red Newsom, Katherine and Greg, Sean Coleman, Linda

Langton, Alice Rees, Karen Ball, Phil Gray, to the lads of Wheeeey, to the Hungry Boys, to the Northern Crime Syndicate, to my FYR brothers and the R007! Family. All have done so much for me, and I'm not sure they know how much I'm thankful.

This industry is incredible at times, and a few people have really shown me kindness that has gone above and beyond. Graham Bartlett, FE Birch, Heather Fitt, Luca Veste, Rob Rutherford, Luca Veste, Craig Robertson, Alexandra Sokoloff, Vaseem Khan and Steve Mosby. My gratitude is endless.

To every reader and bookseller and blogger. The support I've had in my career is giant, and overwhelming. Thank you all so deeply, and you ain't see nothing yet.

Finally, a huge thank you to my agent Maddalena Cavaciuti. Being part of the DHA family is one of the greatest things ever to happen to my career, and I want to thank you all. But Maddalena has changed everything for me, and I do mean everything. In the years we've worked together, she's inspired, galvanised, supported and advised with such passion, skill and potency, that I look at what's happening and know it's to her I owe so much thanks. And just like Therese, I know she'd probably wished I stopped now.

And I'm guessing you, reading this, are ready for me to stop too. But the last one is for you. Thank YOU, for picking up this book. You've no idea how much the fact you're reading this right now blows this writer's mind.

A Note on the Author

ROB PARKER is the author of *Far From the Tree*, the #1 bestselling thriller for Audible Original and the first instalment in the *Thirty Miles* trilogy, as well as eight novels for independent publishers. He is the host of Crime Central Manchester, a monthly showcase of emerging crime writing talent and blockbuster bestsellers. Rob lives in Warrington with his wife, three children and their dogs, and was inspired to write *The Troubled Deep* by years of holidays in the Norfolk Broads – during which he has never, he is pleased to say, found a dead body.

A Note on the Type

The text of this book is set in Bembo, which was first used in 1495 by the Venetian printer Aldus Manutius for Cardinal Bembo's *De Aetna*. The original types were cut for Manutius by Francesco Griffo. Bembo was one of the types used by Claude Garamond (1480–1561) as a model for his Romain de l'Université, and so it was a forerunner of what became the standard European type for the following two centuries. Its modern form follows the original types and was designed for Monotype in 1929.